The International Library of Psychology

THE PRINCIPLES OF TEACHING

Founded by C. K. Ogden

The International Library of Psychology

DEVELOPMENTAL PSYCHOLOGY
In 32 Volumes

I	The Child's Discovery of Death	*Anthony*
II	The Psychology of the Infant	*Bernfeld*
III	The Psychology of Special Abilities and Disabilities	*Bronner*
IV	The Child and His Family	*Bühler*
V	From Birth to Maturity	*Bühler*
VI	The Mental Development of the Child	*Bühler*
VII	The Psychology of Children's Drawings	*Eng*
VIII	Educational Psychology	*Fox*
IX	A Study of Imagination in Early Childhood	*Griffiths*
X	Understanding Children's Play	*Hartley et al*
XI	Intellectual Growth in Young Children	*Isaacs*
XII	Conversations with Children	*Katz*
XIII	The Growth of the Mind	*Koffka*
XIV	The Child's Unconscious Mind	*Lay*
XV	Infant Speech	*Lewis*
XVI	The Growth of Reason	*Lorimer*
XVII	The Growing Child and its Problems	*Miller*
XVIII	The Child's Conception of Physical Causality	*Piaget*
XIX	The Child's Conception of Geometry	*Piaget et al*
XX	The Construction of Reality in the Child	*Piaget*
XXI	The Early Growth of Logic in the Child	*Inhelder et al*
XXII	The Growth of Logical Thinking from Childhood to Adolescence	*Inhelder et al*
XXIII	Judgement and Reasoning in the Child	*Piaget*
XXIV	The Moral Judgment of the Child	*Piaget*
XXV	Play, Dreams and Imitation in Childhood	*Piaget*
XXVI	The Psychology of Intelligence	*Piaget*
XXVII	Mental Health and Infant Development, V1	*Soddy*
XXVIII	Mental Health and Infant Development, V2	*Soddy*
XXIX	Modern Psychology and Education	*Sturt*
XXX	The Dynamics of Education	*Taba*
XXXI	Education Psychology	*Thorndike*
XXXII	The Principles of Teaching	*Thorndike*

THE PRINCIPLES OF TEACHING

Based on Psychology

EDWARD L THORNDIKE

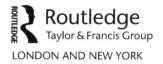

LONDON AND NEW YORK

First published in 1906 by
Routledge and Kegan Paul Ltd.
2 Park Square, Milton Park, Abingdon, Oxfordshire OX14 4RN
711 Third Avenue, New York, NY 10017

First issued in paperback 2014

Routledge is an imprint of the Taylor and Francis Group, an informa business

© 1906 Edward L Thorndike

All rights reserved. No part of this book may be reprinted or reproduced
or utilized in any form or by any electronic, mechanical, or other means,
now known or hereafter invented, including photocopying
and recording, or in any information storage or retrieval system, without
permission in writing from the publishers.

The publishers have made every effort to contact authors/copyright holders
of the works reprinted in the *International Library of Psychology*.
This has not been possible in every case, however, and we would
welcome correspondence from those individuals/companies
we have been unable to trace.

These reprints are taken from original copies of each book. In many cases
the condition of these originals is not perfect. The publisher has gone to
great lengths to ensure the quality of these reprints, but wishes to point
out that certain characteristics of the original copies will, of necessity, be
apparent in reprints thereof.

British Library Cataloguing in Publication Data
A CIP catalogue record for this book
is available from the British Library

The Principles of Teaching
ISBN 0415-21012-7
Developmental Psychology: 32 Volumes
ISBN 0415-21128-X
The International Library of Psychology: 204 Volumes
ISBN 0415-19132-7

ISBN 13: 978-1-138-87520-3 (pbk)
ISBN 13: 978-0-415-21012-6 (hbk)

PREFACE

The aim of this book is to make the study of teaching scientific and practical—scientific in the sense of dealing with verifiable facts rather than attractive opinions, practical in the sense of giving knowledge and power that will make a difference in the actual work of teaching. It follows the example of the better books on education in basing principles of teaching upon the laws of psychology; it makes use of modern scientific psychology and especially of recent investigations in genetic and dynamic psychology; it seeks to make use also of the direct studies of teaching itself which have been made by qualified experts; it is arranged as a manual to guide the student in applying principles himself rather than as a series of discussions to be thought out or, more often, to be simply absorbed.

The book demands of students knowledge of the elements of psychology, particularly of dynamic psychology. The references entitled 'Preparatory' (or their equivalent) will fulfill this prerequisite. These references are to the author's *Elements of Psychology,* which is in a sense an introduction to the present volume, but any standard course in psychology which gives due emphasis to the laws of mental connections will supply the preparation needed.

Scientific principles are the back-bone of knowledge of teaching but concrete exercises are its flesh and blood. For the work of the student of teaching is to get practical control of principles by using them. The author offers no excuse for using over a third of his pages for such vi *Preface*

exercises; indeed, they should occupy more than two-thirds of the student's time. They aim in some cases to test and increase the student's knowledge of principles; in others to insure the habit and power of application of general principles to the particular problems of the school-room; in others to give training in judging the theories, methods and devices which each year's output of educational literature brings to a teacher's attention. In all cases they aim to make thought about teaching more logical and scientific.

The references for further reading are of two sorts. The first, given at the end of each chapter, are to readings designed to extend the knowledge given in the text or to suggest useful comparisons. These readings are all included in ten books so chosen as to give students an adequate view of the present status of knowledge and expert opinion about teaching, and to form the nucleus of a teacher's professional library. They are:—

J. Adams, *The Herbartian Psychology Applied to Education,* 1898.[1]

A. Bain, *Education as a Science,* 1887.

J. Dewey, *School and Society,* 1900.

C. W. Eliot, *Educational Reform,* 1898

E. W. Hope and E. A. Browne, *A Manual of School Hygiene,* 1901.

W. James, *Talks to Teachers on Psychology,* 1899.

E. A. Kirkpatrick, *The Fundamentals of Child Study,* 1903.

J. MacCunn, *The Making of Character,* 1900.

C. A. McMurry and F. M. McMurry, *The Method of the Recitation* (revised edition), 1903.

---

[1] The dates give the edition to which the reference applies. Any edition will serve, however, except in the case of the McMurrys' Method of the Recitation, where the edition should be 1903 or later.

Preface vii

H. Spencer, *Education: Intellectual, Moral, and Physical* (the references fit any edition).

The second sort of references, given at the end of the book, are designed to aid students in such studies of special topics as they may profitably undertake.

In the text there are ninety-seven quotations, mostly of passages requiring critical comment in the *Exercises.* Since the student should in such cases make his judgments uninfluenced by the source of the passage, the sources are not given in the text. For the sake of anyone who may need to know the source of any such quotation a number in brackets follow each and, in the SOURCES OF QUOTATIONS at the end of the book, the reference is given for each number. When it is proper that the source of a quotation should be known at the time that it is read, the reference is given in the text itself also.

Teachers College, Columbia University,
December, 1905.

CONTENTS

CHAPTER I
INTRODUCTION

§ 1. *The Teacher's Problem*............................ 1
§ 2. *Psychology and the Art of Teaching* 7
§ 3. *Exercises* 10

CHAPTER II
PHYSICAL EDUCATION

§ 4. *The Care of the Body*............................ 12
§ 5. *Remedying Defects*................................ 14
§ 6. *The Prevention of Defects*........................ 16
§ 7. *Exercises* 17

CHAPTER III
INSTINCTS AND CAPACITIES

§ 8. *Natural Tendencies in General*...................... **21**
§ 9. *Instincts* 24
§ 10. *Capacities* 29
§ 11. *Exercises* 34
§ 12. *Self-Activity* 39

CHAPTER IV
APPERCEPTION

§ 13. *The General Law*.............................. 42
§ 14. *Detailed Applications: Exercises*.................... 43

CHAPTER V
INTERESTS

§ 15. *The Meaning of Interests*.......................... 51
§ 16. *Interests as Ends*................................ 52
§ 17. *Interests as Means*................................ 54
§ 18. *Exercises* 59

x   *Contents*

CHAPTER VI
INDIVIDUAL DIFFERENCES

§ 19. *Variability in General* 68
§ 20. *Differences in General Mental Constitution* 85
§ 21. *Differences in Thought* 87
§ 22. *Differences in Action* 92
§ 23. *Differences in Temperament* 94
§ 24. *Sex Differences* 96
§ 25. *Exercises* 98

CHAPTER VII
ATTENTION

§ 26. *Instinct and Habit and Attention* 105
§ 27. *Exercises* 107

CHAPTER VIII
PRINCIPLES OF ASSOCIATION

§ 28. *Habit Formation* 110
§ 29. *Exercises* 112
§ 30. *Memory* 123
§ 31. *Exercises* 124
§ 32. *Correlation* 127
§ 33. *Exercises* 129

CHAPTER IX
PRINCIPLES OF ANALYSIS

§ 34. *Principles of Teaching* 133
§ 35. *Their Application: Exercises* 135

CHAPTER X
REASONING

§ 36. *Reasoning as Selective Thinking* 147
§ 37. *Inductive Methods of Teaching* 154
§ 38. *Deductive Methods of Teaching* 160
§ 39. *Exercises* 164

Contents **xi**

CHAPTER XI
RESPONSES OF CONDUCT: MORAL TRAINING

§ 40. *Education and Conduct*.............................. 179
§ 41. *School Habits as Moral Training*................... 185
§ 42. *Specific Moral Instruction*........................ 187
§ 43. *The Moral Effects of School Studies*................ 189
§ 44. *Exercises* 194

CHAPTER XII
RESPONSES OF FEELING

§ 45. *The Real Emotions*................................. 198
§ 46. *The Aesthetic Emotions*............................ 200
§ 47. *Exercises* 202

CHAPTER XIII
MOTOR EXPRESSION

§ 48. *The Relation of Motor Responses to Thought and Feeling* 206
§ 49. *Verbal Expression*................................. 208
§ 50. *The Activities of the Arts and Industries*............. 210
§ 51. *Dangers to be Avoided*............................. 212
§ 52. *Exercises* 215

CHAPTER XIV
MOTOR EDUCATION

§ 53. *Teaching Form*.................................... 219
§ 54. *Teaching Execution*................................ 222
§ 55. *Exercises* 228

CHAPTER XV
FORMAL DISCIPLINE

§ 56. *The Superstition of General Training*................ 235
§ 57. *The Specialization of Abilities*.................... 238
§ 58. *The Amount of Influence of Special Training*......... 240
§ 59. *The Method of Influence of Special Training*........ 243
§ 60. *Exercises* 249

xii *Contents*

CHAPTER XVI

THE SCIENTIFIC STUDY OF TEACHING

§ 61. *Testing the Results of Teaching*.......... 257
§ 62. *Testing the General Results of School Work*.......... 264
§ 63. *A Typical Scientific Study of School Work*........... 268

TOPICS FOR FURTHER STUDY, WITH REFERENCES.... 274

SOURCES OF QUOTATIONS........................ 281

INDEX OF EXERCISES RELATING TO SPECIAL SCHOOL
SUBJECTS 286

INDEX OF EXPERIMENTS........................ 287

INDEX OF SUBJECTS............................ 288

The Principles of Teaching

CHAPTER I

INTRODUCTION

§ 1. *The Teacher's Problem*

The Aims, Materials and Methods of Education.— The word Education is used with many meanings, but in all its usages it refers to *changes*. No one is educated who stays just as he was. We do not educate anybody if we do nothing that makes any difference or change in anybody. The need of education arises from the fact that *what is* is not what *ought to be*. Because we wish ourselves and others to become different from what we and they now are, we try to educate ourselves and them. In studying education, then, one studies always the existence, nature, causation or value of changes of some sort.

The teacher confronts two questions: 'What changes to make?' and 'How to make them?' The first question is commonly answered for the teacher by the higher school authorities for whom he or she works. The opinions of the educational leaders in the community decide what the schools shall try to do for their pupils. The program of studies is planned and the work which is to be done grade by grade is carefully outlined. The grammar-school teacher may think that changes in knowledge represented by the ability to read a modern language ought to be made in boys and girls before the high-school, but the decision is rarely his; the primary

2 The Principles of Teaching

teacher may be obliged to teach arithmetic although her own judgment would postpone giving the knowledge of numbers until the fifth or sixth grade.

What changes should be made in human nature by primary, grammar and high schools and why these and not other changes should be the aim of the schools, are questions usually answered under the heading of 'Principles of Education.' How most efficiently to make such changes as educational aims recommend, is a question usually answered under the headings 'Principles of Teaching,' or 'Methods of Teaching,' or 'Theory and Practice of Teaching,' or 'Educational Psychology.' This book will try to answer this latter question,—to give a scientific basis for the art of actual teaching rather than for the selection of aims for the schools as a whole or of the subjects to be taught or of the general result to be gained from any subject. Not the *What* or the *Why* but the *How* is its topic.

It is not wise however to study the *How* of teaching without any reference to the *What* or the *Why*. If a teacher does not appreciate, at least crudely, the general aims of education, he will not fully appreciate the general aims of school education; if he does not appreciate the general aims of school education, he will not fully appreciate the aims of his special grade or of any one special subject; if he does not have fairly clear ideas of what the year's work as a whole or of what each subject as a whole ought to accomplish for the scholars, he will not know exactly what he is about in any particular day's work. The teacher must be something more than the carpenter who follows without reflection the architect's plan, or the nurse who merely administers the physician's prescriptions. His relation to the administration of the school system and the program of studies is more like that

Introduction 3

of the builder who is told to make the best house he can at a cost of ten thousand dollars, using three laborers, a derrick and such and such tools and providing especially for light, ventilation and protection against fire. Superior authorities say, 'Make the best boys and girls you can, using arithmetic, geography, school regulations and so on, providing especially for knowledge, good habits of thought, worthy interests, bodily health, noble feelings and honest, unselfish conduct.' The builder must often study how to dig a foundation, how to erect a frame, how to lay a floor and the like with reference to what is to be built; the teacher should often study how to utilize inborn tendencies, how to form habits, how 'to develop interests and the like with reference to what changes in intellect and character are to be made. The teacher should know about educational aims and values as well as about such principles of teaching as directly concern his own activities in the class-room.

The next three pages will accordingly outline the essential facts concerning the ideals which, in the opinion of the best qualified thinkers, should be followed in American education, and throughout the book due attention will be given to such facts about the ends the teacher should seek as he needs to know to improve his teaching.

The Aims of Education.—Education as a whole should make human beings wish each other well, should increase the sum of human energy and happiness and decrease the sum of discomfort of the human beings that are or will be, and should foster the higher, impersonal pleasures. These aims of education in general—good-will to men, useful and happy lives, and noble enjoyment—are the ultimate aims of school education in particular. Its proximate aims are to give boys and girls health in body and mind, information about the world of nature

4 *The Principles of Teaching*

and men, worthy interests in knowledge and action, a multitude of habits of thought, feeling and behavior and ideals of efficiency, honor, duty, love and service. The special proximate aims of the first six years of school life are commonly taken to be to give physical training and protection against disease; knowledge of the simple facts of nature and human life; the ability to gain knowledge and pleasure through reading and to express ideas and feelings through spoken and written language, music and other arts; interests in the concrete life of the world; habits of intelligent curiosity, purposive thinking, modesty, obedience, honesty, helpfulness, affection, courage and justice; and the ideals proper to childhood.

The special proximate aims of school life from twelve to eighteen are commonly taken to be physical health and skill; knowledge of the simpler general laws of nature and human life and of the opinions of the wisest and best; more effective use of the expressive arts; interests in the arts and sciences, and in human life both as directly experienced and as portrayed in literature; powers of self-control, accuracy, steadiness and logical thought, technical and executive abilities, cooperation and leadership; habits of self-restraint, honor, courage, justice, sympathy and reverence; and the ideals proper to youth.

With respect to the amount of emphasis upon different features of these general ideals, the best judgment of the present rates practical ability somewhat higher and culture of the semi-selfish sort somewhat lower than has been the case in the past. No sensible thinker about education now regards the ability to support oneself as a mean thing. Every one must gain power at school as well as at home to pull his own weight in the boat, to repay in useful labor what the world gives him in food and shelter. The cultured idler is as one-sided as the

Introduction 5

ignorant and clownish worker and may be even more of a danger to the world. The schools must prepare for efficiency in the serious business of life as well as for the refined enjoyment of its leisure.

The best judgment of the present gives much more weight than has been the case previously to health, to bodily skill and to the technical and industrial arts. The ideal of the scholar has given way to the ideal of the capable man,—capable in scholarship still, but also capable in physique and in the power to manipulate things.

Very recently thinkers about education have dwelt more and more upon the importance of aiming not only to prepare children for adult life and work but also to adapt them to the life of childhood itself. Aim more to make children succeed with the problems and duties of childhood and less to fit them for the problems and duties of twenty years after; let education adapt the child to his own environment as well as to some supposed work of his later years—such are the recommendations of present-day theories of education.

In actual practice aims often conflict. A gain in knowledge may mean a loss in health; to arouse ideals may mean less time for drill in correct habits; in zeal for the development of love of the beautiful the interest in the dry, cold facts of science may have to be neglected. The energy of any teacher, and of scholars as well, is limited. All that can be expected is that none of the aims of school education shall be wilfully violated and that energy should be distributed among them all in some reasonable way.

The degrees of emphasis on the different proximate aims vary (1) with the nature of the individual to be educated and (2) with the nature of the educational forces besides the school which are at work. Thus (1) the

6 *The Principles of Teaching*

emphasis in a school for the feeble-minded is not the same as in an ordinary school; the emphasis in a high school representing a selection of the more ambitious, intellectual and energetic is not the same as in a school where the selection is simply on the basis of the ability of the parents to pay tuition. (2) The emphasis in a primary school attended by the children of recent immigrants will differ from that in a school in a suburb inhabited by American professional and business families. A high school in a farming community in the Southwest should not pattern its ideals after those proper to a school in New York City.

The Special Problem of the Teacher.—It is the problem of the higher authorities of the schools to decide what the schools shall try to achieve and to arrange plans for school work which will attain the desired ends. Having decided what changes are to be made they entrust to the teachers the work of making them. The special problem of the teacher is to make these changes as economically and as surely as is possible under the conditions of school life. His is the task of giving certain information, forming certain habits, increasing certain powers, arousing certain interests and inspiring certain ideals.

The study of the best methods of doing so may be carried to almost any degree of detail. The principles of teaching may mean the general principles applicable to the formation of all habits or the highly specialized rules of procedure for forming the habit of correct use of *shall* and *will;* they include the laws valid for the acquisition of any knowledge and the discussion of the particular difficulties in teaching the spelling of *to, two* and *too*. But the problem is always fundamentally the same:— Given these children to be changed and this change to be made, how shall I proceed? Given this material for

Introduction 7

education and this aim of education, what means and methods shall I use?

§ 2. *Psychology and the Art of Teaching*

The Scientific Basis of Teaching.—The work of teaching is to produce and to prevent changes in human beings; to preserve and increase the desirable qualities of body, intellect and character and to get rid of the undesirable. To thus control human nature, the teacher needs to know it. To change what is into what ought to be, we need to know the laws by which the changes occur. Just as to make a plant grow well the gardener must act in accordance with the laws of botany which concern the growth of plants, or as to make a bridge well the architect must act in accordance with the facts of mechanics concerning stresses and strains, or as to change disease into health the physician must act in accordance with the laws of physiology and pathology, so to make human beings intelligent and useful and noble the teacher must act in accordance with the laws of the sciences of human nature.

The sciences of biology, especially human physiology and hygiene, give the laws of changes in bodily nature. The science of psychology gives the laws of changes in intellect and character. The teacher studies and learns to apply psychology to teaching for the same reason that the progressive farmer studies and learns to apply botany; the architect, mechanics; or the physician, physiology and pathology.

Stimulus and Response.—Using psychological terms, the art of teaching may be defined as the art of giving and withholding stimuli with the result of producing or preventing certain responses. In this definition the term stimulus is used widely for any event which

8   *The Principles of Teaching*

influences a person,—for a word spoken to him, a look, a sentence which he reads, the air he breathes, etc., etc. The term response is used for any reaction made by him, —a new thought, a feeling of interest, a bodily act, any mental or bodily condition resulting from the stimulus. The aim of the teacher is to produce desirable and prevent undesirable changes in human beings by producing and preventing certain responses. The means at the disposal of the teacher are the stimuli which can be brought to bear upon the pupil,—the teacher's words, gestures and appearance, the condition and appliances of the school room, the books to be used and objects to be seen, and so on through a long list of the things and events which the teacher can control. The responses of the pupil· are all the infinite variety of thoughts and feelings and bodily movements occurring in all their possible connections.

The stimuli given by the teacher to arouse and guide the pupil's responses may be classified as:—

A. Stimuli under direct control.

   The teacher's movements,[1]—speech, gestures, facial expression, etc.

B. Stimuli under indirect control.

   The physical conditions of the school,—air, light, heat, etc.

   The material equipment of the school,— books, apparatus, specimens, etc.

   The social conditions of the school,—the acts (including spoken words) of the pupils and the spirit which these acts represent.

   The general environment,—acts of parents, laws, libraries, etc.

[1] The knowledge, love and tact of the teacher are, of course, of the highest importance as forces in teaching but their actual operation is in their expression in words, gestures or acts of some sort.

Introduction 9

The responses may be classified as:—

A. Physiological responses, such as deeper breathing, sounder sleep, vigorous exercise and the like.

B. Responses of knowledge,[1] such as connecting a sense stimulus with an appropriate percept, abstracting one element from a complex fact or making associations of ideas.

C. Responses of attitude, such as the connection of attention, interest, preference and belief with certain situations.

D. Responses of feeling, such as connecting sympathy, love, hate, etc., with certain situations.

E. Responses of action or of conduct and skill, connecting certain acts or movements with certain mental states.

The Value of Psychology.—If there existed a perfect and complete knowledge of human nature,—a complete science of psychology,—it would tell the effect of every possible stimulus and the cause of every possible response in every possible human being. A teacher could then know just what the result of any act of his would be, could prophesy just what the effect of such and such a page read or punishment given or dress worn would be,—just how to get any particular response, of attention to this object, memory of this fact or comprehension of that principle.

Of course present knowledge of psychology is nearer to zero than to complete perfection, and its applications to teaching must therefore be often incomplete, indefinite and insecure. The application of psychology to teaching is more like that of botany and chemistry to farming than like that of physiology and pathology to medicine.

[1] Knowledge is used here in a broad sense to include sensing objects, analyzing facts, feeling relationships and drawing inferences, as well as memory of facts or associations of ideas.

10 *The Principles of Teaching*

Anyone of good sense can farm fairly well without science, and anyone of good sense can teach fairly well without knowing and applying psychology. Still, as the farmer with the knowledge of the applications of botany and chemistry to farming is, other things being equal, more successful than the farmer without it, so the teacher will, other things being equal, be the more successful who can apply psychology, the science of human nature, to the problems of the school.

§ 3. *Exercises*

1. In teaching which of the following subjects would you depend most upon responses of knowledge? Upon responses of feeling? Upon responses of action?—Literature, manual training, Latin.

2. Rank the following subjects in order according to the importance in them of responses of analysis: Music, History, Grammar.

3. Rank them according to the importance of responses of feeling.

4. Name two school studies which specially seek responses of observation.

5. Name two which specially seek responses of bodily skill.

6. Name two which specially seek responses of inference.

7. What sort of response is implied in each of the following?

> a. Learning the meanings of the numbers from one to seven.
> b. Learning to dance.
> c.   "   to love one's enemies.
> d.   "   the definition of a verb.

Introduction 11

e. Learning the sounds of the letters.

f. " to obey a teacher.

g. " the principal parts of a verb.

h. " to study in a noisy room.

i. " to be good-natured, though provoked.

8. To teach some of the school subjects, one must call forth responses of all four kinds, of knowledge, attitude, feeling and action. Show that this statement is true of geography.

9. Name some stimuli besides words and books which are essential in teaching geography.

10. In teaching morality.

11. In promoting the enjoyment of school life.

12. In training for good citizenship.

For Further Reading

C. W. Eliot, *Educational Reform,* Chapters III, V-XIV inclusive, and XVIII.

H. Spencer, *Education,* Chapter I.

J. Adams, *Herbartian Psychology Applied to Education,* Chapters I and II.

CHAPTER II

PHYSICAL EDUCATION

§ 4. *The Care of the Body*

As an End in Itself.—Bodily health and vigor are important in education both as ends and as means. They are ends because happiness and usefulness depend upon a sound body as well as upon a sound mind and morals. The school must accept a share with the home and with private and public agencies of the burden of maintaining the natural vigor of children, preventing diseases and remedying defects. It is its duty to keep children's eyes in good condition as well as to teach them to read. To prevent scarlet fever or to eradicate consumption is the duty of the school as well as of the hospital. The teacher must teach for health as well as for knowledge or conduct, and the well-equipped teacher will know and apply physiology and hygiene.

The special principles of physical education lie outside the scope of this book. But some very general rules of guidance may be stated.

Health is better than strength or grace. The action of the heart and other parts of the circulatory system, of the lungs, of the digestive organs and of the excretory organs is far more important than the action of the voluntary muscles of arms, legs and chest. The indirect results of exercise upon the system in general outweigh tenfold the direct effect on the size and strength of the muscles.

Physical Education 13

Pure air, nourishing food and sound sleep are the essentials for healthy growth. Exercise is probably essential also, but no system of gymnastics can make up for a lack in the other three. As a rule free movements, such as swimming, are superior to forced movements involving sudden inhibitions and opposing contractions. such as the common dumb-bell drills. Exercise outdoors is better than exercise in any ordinary gymnasium and far better than exercise in a school class-room. Exercise taken in play with enjoyment is better than exercise taken as a task.

As a Means to Intellectual and Moral Welfare.— Under present conditions the class-room teacher, though concerned with bodily health as an aim of the school, is perhaps more concerned with bodily conditions as means to the production of desirable changes in intellect and character. For the mind is the servant of the body as well as its master, and the mind's responses are often best influenced through bodily conditions. For example, the quality of the work of a primary-school class may be raised several degrees by the proper seating of children who are partially deaf and by the provision of proper glasses for children with defects of vision. The general efficiency of the vital organs is the desirable if not the necessary basis for good spirits, good conduct and good thinking. For the sake of proper intellectual and moral progress, then, as well as for the sake of the health and happiness of the scholars, teachers should cooperate with families and public agencies in remedying and preventing defects and in improving general bodily conditions.

The relation between bodily conditions and mental welfare is not everywhere equally close. The loss of one's toes makes little difference, whereas the loss of one's eyes is an enormous handicap. Pneumonia rarely, but

14   *The Principles of Teaching*

scarlet fever often, leaves mental weakness in its train. Strength of an arm means little to either intellect or disposition, but skill of hand and eye is a great aid in school work. A good digestion is the mother of cheerfulness and peace. As a rule what influences the central nervous system, the organs of sense and the nervous and muscular apparatus for moving the eyes, mouth-parts and hands, will have a direct effect upon intellectual activities.

§ 5. *Remedying Defects*

Defects of Sight and Hearing.—Unless the stimuli given by the teacher are properly felt, proper responses cannot be made. ·No matter how cleverly the teacher talks, it will be vain unless the pupil hears. Knowledge that a child has only one-tenth of normal acuity of vision may be of greater help in teaching him than many elaborate books and pictures.

There will rarely be a class of thirty scholars without two or more children who have defects of vision or hearing so great as to seriously impair their power of receiving stimuli. If the pupils so affected were themselves conscious of their defects, not so much harm would be done; but in point of fact college students are found who are totally deaf in one ear or blind in one eye or markedly color blind without being in the least aware of it, and in the first years of school life a large proportion of the children defective in hearing or vision are entirely unaware of their difficulty. The deaf ones have for so long had to strain every nerve and watch people's gestures and half guess at the meaning of the dimly and partially heard words that they have no reason to think of their condition as anything peculiar. Those defective in vision have for so long been obliged to labor to decipher and

Physical Education 15

interpret the misty, fleeting objects of vision,—reading has so commonly meant a headache to them,—that they take their troubles as a matter of course. Young children cannot be expected to themselves discover and report their defects; their parents will often do as little. The school must not only give proper stimuli but also note the condition of the organs for receiving stimuli, remedying the defects which exist when possible, and so arranging the class instruction that irremediable defects will do the least possible harm.

Other Defects. Gross defects of the motor apparatus such as paralyses and contractures, are fairly obvious; common sense as well as psychology will recommend that allowance be made for pupils suffering from them in the work of writing, drawing and the like.

Obstruction of the throat and nasal passages by enlarged tonsils and adenoid growths is a not uncommon cause of deafness and dullness. Teachers should observe carefully any children who habitually breathe through the mouth and should cooperate with parents to secure medical advice for them. In many cases the safe and easy operation of removing such growths brings a marked improvement in the comfort and school progress of the pupil.

Within the last decade the schools have more and more extended the work of cooperating with the family and public authorities with respect to the care of other bodily defects. Some school systems provide for an examination of the children's teeth and for securing necessary dental work; some send trained nurses to the houses to instruct parents in the treatment of minor diseases. It has been proposed to establish special schools for cripples.

Teachers may feel sure that their cooperation with

16   *The Principles of Teaching*

any wise plan for the amelioration of physical defects will result not only in improving the physical health of the community but also in making more efficient the intellectual and moral training of the school. It may not seem to be, and may not be, the teacher's business to cure a toothache, but there may be no more effective way to insure a pupil's progress than to get rid of the physical pain, the digestive disorders, the eye troubles and the susceptibility to diseases of the throat which may result from decayed teeth.

§ 6. *The Prevention of Defects*

All the arguments for the cure of defects apply with even greater force to their prevention. Schools should be positive forces for health and teachers should study and practice the requirements of school hygiene, not only because health should be an aim of the school but also because health is a means to mental and moral welfare.

Unfortunately there is in some respects a conflict between the demands of health and the demands of intellectual and moral training. There would probably be fewer eye troubles if we never read books or worked at occupations demanding skill; children would probably be less sickly if till the age of sixteen they spent the twenty-five hours a week of school time in running, swimming, play with animals, and work out of doors in garden, field and woods. To some extent we barter our health for the other valuables,—knowledge, skill, and habits of utility to the community. At present we probably thus sell too much of health, but it would be equally unwise to sacrifice everything for health. It is better to be a Socrates with a headache than a perfectly healthy pig. There must be a compromise.

Physical Education 17

At all events, it is idiotic to neglect health when its neglect means mental and moral loss also; it is wicked to sacrifice it for nothing; and it is unwise not to rank its claims as approximately equal to those of the intellect.

General Bodily Conditions.—The teacher can only to a slight extent control the air, light, food, sleep and exercise of a class. The large size of classes, the character of school buildings and grounds, the five-sixths of the pupil's time that are spent away from the school and many other factors limit the teacher's influence. But when half of the six-year-olds in a primary class come to school after a breakfast of two or three bakehouse cakes and a cup of coffee or with none, it is a question whether the teacher had not better give up a week to teaching the parents rather than the children. In some city kindergartens it would be better for half the children to be put to bed than set to play.

SUMMARY

Good teaching treats health as of importance comparable with intellectual progress. Good teaching takes account of the bodily conditions of pupils and cooperates with parents and public authorities for their improvement.

The teacher should first, know these bodily conditions in the case of each pupil; second, do what is appropriate to remedy them; and third, allow for them in arrangements for teaching and in estimates of pupils.

§ 7. Exercises

1. What is your opinion of each of the following facts?

(a) In a city school seventy per cent. of the pupils spent over five hours a day (except on Saturdays and

18   *The Principles of Teaching*

Sundays) in home work in preparation of school lessons, and less than an hour and a half a day outdoors.

(b) A nine-year-old boy was inattentive and very restless in school; his teacher rebuked him and he complained of having a headache; his teacher paid no attention to his complaint and on further misbehavior on his part sent him to the principal for punishment; the principal took his temperature, found it to be over 102 and sent him home, with a note for his parents.

2. What would you have written in the note to the parents?

3. Make out a set of rules such as you think a teacher ought to follow with respect to the health regulations of the city in which he or she lives, to acquaintance with free clinics and the means of admission to them, to medical inspectors of schools, to knowledge of the ventilating system of the school building and to the examination of vision and hearing.

4. What do boys and girls commonly buy for luncheon when because of the length of the session or for other reasons they do eat a luncheon at school?

5. Make out (a) a list of five or more articles of food which you would require to be on sale in a school lunch room; (b) a list of five or more articles of food which you would not allow to be sold.

6. Illustrate the fact that a little knowledge may be a dangerous thing by causing a teacher to attempt the work properly belonging to a physician.

7. Illustrate the fact that true care for the health of children does not mean constant inquiry about their symptoms or advice to them about their habits.

8. What measures besides reseating can you devise to assist a deaf pupil?

Physical Education 19

9. What measures can you devise to assist a near-sighted pupil besides fitting him with proper glasses?

10. Very little children when reading often hold their books only partly open, say at an angle of 100 instead of 180 degrees. Should primers and other beginning books be stiffly bound? Should they have the wider margin on the inner or the outer edge of the page?

11. Name three studies in which color blindness would injure a pupil's work.

12. Why would it be important to know of physical defects even though nothing could be done to cure them or to make the pupil work more easily in spite of them?

13. Name two or more features of high-school work which involve an extra tax on the eyes with little compensating value (*e. g.*, the use of German print).

Experiment 1. Record the time taken by six or eight children, to read passage A. To read passage B. Record their answers to the question, 'Which is the easier to read?' What conclusions do you draw concerning blackboard writing and the printing of school-books?

A.

I mused for some time upon what he had said, and found it was a very rational conclusion, and that therefore something was to be resolved on very speedily, as well to draw the men on board into some snare for their surprise, as to prevent their landing upon us, and destroying us; upon this it presently occurred to me, that in a little while, the ship's crew, wondering what was become of their comrades, and of the boat, would certainly come on shore in their other boat to seek for them; and that then perhaps they might come armed, and be too strong for us: this he allowed was rational. Upon this I told him, the first thing we were to do, was to stave the boat, which lay upon the beach, so that they might not carry her off: and taking everything out of her, leave her so far useless as not

20 *The Principles of Teaching*

B.

It was happy for the poor man that it was my man Friday; for he, having been used to that kind of creature in his country, had no fear upon him, but went close up to him, and shot him as above; whereas any of us would have fired at a further distance, and have perhaps either missed the wolf, or endangered shooting the man. But it was enough to have terrified a bolder man than I, and indeed it alarmed all our company, when, with the noise of Friday's pistol, we heard on both sides the dismallest howlings of wolves, and the noise redoubled by the echo of the mountains, that it was to us as if there had been a prodigious multitude of them ; and perhaps indeed there was not such a few, as that we had no cause of apprehensions. However, as Friday had killed this wolf, the other, that had fastened upon the horse, left him immediately, and fled having happily fastened upon his head,

For Further Reading

E. W. Hope and E. A. Browne, *A Manual of School Hygiene,* Chapters III-XIV inclusive.

E. A. Kirkpatrick, *Fundamentals of Child Study,* Chapter XVII.

CHAPTER III

INSTINCTS AND CAPACITIES

Preparatory, *Elements of Psychology,* §§ 30-34[1]

§ 8. *Natural Tendencies in General*

What human beings become depends upon the tendencies which are born in them as well as the training which is given to them. Nature as well as nurture forms human intellect and character. To be effective, nurture or education must allow for the forces of nature. To teach boys and girls without paying heed to the equipment of instincts and capacities which they already possess apart from teaching would be as foolish as to sail a boat regardless of the direction of the wind or to build a house regardless of the material at hand.

Education should at times stimulate and favor inborn tendencies, at times inhibit them, and, most frequently of all, direct and guide them. The capacity for active thought and reasoning, for instance, needs encouragement; the teasing and bullying instinct must be inhibited; the inborn tendencies to curiosity and sympathy must be directed into useful channels and transformed into habits of intelligent thinking or sensible and noble action. Mere greed of knowledge is of value only in its possibilities; to pity everything and everybody may be as truly a vice as to pity no one.

[1] The author's *Elements of Psychology* is the book referred to here and in later preparatory references.

22　　*The Principles of Teaching*

Utilizing Natural Tendencies.—Education may also be made more and more economical in proportion as it utilizes the forces of natural tendencies to attain its ideal ends. Whenever we work with rather than against nature the task becomes easy and the burden light. Fractions become easy with the help of apples and blocks and knives and jig-saw because the instinctive tendencies to attend to concrete objects and to enjoy physical action and manipulation are called into service.

Teaching may be wasteful or even harmful by neglect of the fact of delayed instincts and capacities. Theology for the ten-year-old in Sunday schools and Jane Austen's novels for high-school boys are much the same as cabbage for babies. Cabbage is a good food only when the capacity to digest it exists. Teaching little girls to be attentive to their dress and appearance is much the same as trying to teach an infant of six months to walk. The interest in clothes and looks will come of itself with adolescence just as the walking instinct will come of itself at the beginning of the second year.

Just as the delayed appearance of inborn tendencies makes too early teaching wasteful, so their transitoriness makes too tardy teaching fruitless. The manual dexterity of the pianist, for instance, must be acquired early in life if at all. The instincts and capacities important in education are, however, for the most part long-lived, and, if not suppressed by actual ill-treatment, persist through the years of school life without special stimulation from teachers. So with the instincts of action, curiosity, the love of outdoor life and sport, emulation and many others.

Destroying Natural Tendencies.—Harmful instincts and capacities are weakened or inhibited by *disuse* (by depriving them of exercise, by not allowing the situations which would evoke them to appear), *substitution* (by

Instincts and Capacities

forming the habit of meeting the situation in some other way) and by *punishment*. Thus the tendency of a child to chase and torment a kitten may be inhibited by giving the child no kitten to play with, or by teaching him early to stroke and feed the kitten, or by beating him in case he does pull its tail and throw stones at it.

Disuse is convenient and is an excellent method to employ when the harmful tendency is transitory, but it is never quite sure. *Punishment* is ineffective in the case of very strong instincts. To be of service in any case, it must be so administered as to connect the discomfort closely with the harmful act. *Substitution* is in most cases by far the best method for the teacher's use. Habits of care for pets are the best preventive of cruelty to animals; to divide a class into two groups and give marks to the groups instead of to individuals,—to substitute, that is, team emulation for individual emulation,—may be the best cure for selfish ambition and envy; for a restless class manual work is better than scolding.

Some instincts apparently injurious may have bound up with them valuable traits of intellect and character, and consequently may require encouragement and especially redirection. The annoying questioning of very young children is part and parcel of a general intellectual impulse that is a chief source of mental growth; the disobedience and defiance of boys in their teens, often very troublesome to school and family life, is to some extent at least a necessary accompaniment of the general instinct of independence and mastery which comes at adolescence and which is essential to vigorous manhood; awkwardness and lack of courtesy may be necessary features of a modesty which would suffer if they were artificially overcome.

Individual Differences.—Since individuals differ in

24　The Principles of Teaching

the nature and amounts of their capacities and instincts, the particular equipment of each boy or girl, as well as the general fund possessed by human beings as a species, must be allowed for by the teacher. The general capacity for response to visual stimuli gives reason for the tremendous use of visual stimuli in teaching, but if a boy is blind, the right in general becomes wrong in particular. The general instinct of physical activity recommends constructive work, motor expression and the actual manipulation of objects as means of training for almost all young children; but for the few who are relatively lacking in this instinct and possess in abundance the capacity for abstract thought and pure mental gymnastics, the more scientific and intellectual study of objects and ideas and symbols may be better.

Many responses of attitude as well as of action are instinctive; *e. g.*, the interest of babies in living animals, the interests of adolescents in the opposite sex, the general tendency to attend to the novel and the general interest in achievement. These instincts of interest are hard to separate from instincts of action and could well be discussed in connection with them. From the point of view of their application to teaching, however, it is better to describe them in connection with interests in general in Chapter V.

§ 9. *Instincts*

The following instincts are of special importance in school education:—

Mental Activity,—the tendency to be thinking in some way or another, to avoid mental apathy.

Curiosity,—a special aspect of the instinct of general mental activity; the tendency to provoke ideas, especially in the presence of new situations.

Instincts and Capacities 25

Physical Activity,—the tendency to be doing something, to avoid bodily torpor.

Manipulation,—a special aspect of the instinct of general physical activity; the tendency to handle objects, to move them, take them apart, re-unite them, etc., etc.

Collecting.

Ownership.

Sociability.

Emulation.

Kindliness.

Pugnacity and *Mastery.*

Independence and *Defiance.*

Mental Activity.— The instinct of general mental activity is the fountain head of human intellectual development and has been in the past the chief support of school education. Unlike almost all other animals, man thinks not only under the stress of some immediate practical need, but at all times and for the mere enjoyment of thinking,—thinks not only about the few particular objects that feed, warm, protect or injure him, but about everything he experiences. The kitten's intellect restricts itself to certain smells, sounds and sights that concern food, hunting, play, sleep and the like, and commonly thinks of these only when it is immediately profitable for it to do so. The child watches and listens to all sorts of objects even when they have no meaning for his bodily needs. For to the human being intellectual life is as truly a need as food or safety.

Children do not have to be enticed or forced to think and learn. They seek ideas as eagerly as food. Only when it involves restraint, monotony and futility, is thinking objectionable. The teacher's problem is to preserve the force of the original instinct of mental activity by giving it exercise and by rewarding its exercise with

26 *The Principles of Teaching*

satisfaction, and to guide the aimless, random thinking of children into useful and rational forms.

The greater part of the imitative play of children is a result of this instinct of general mental activity. Playing father, mother, grocer, automobile, church, school and the like is an easy means of arousing trains of thought without strain or fatigue. The amount that children teach each other in the course of such free play is a witness to the value of the instinct and should be a lesson to every teacher.

Physical Activity.—The instinct of general physical activity with its special form, the manipulation of objects,[1] is the original source of sports, industries and arts, and is in childhood the prime ally of intellectual development. As children think for the sake of thinking, so also they move about and handle objects just for the love of action and of the new ideas which action brings. The dog does a few things to a small variety of objects and can become a hunter, eater and carrier; the child does all sorts of things to almost everything and can become a talker, writer, carpenter, violinist and hundreds of things besides.

One aim of the school is to direct the force that makes children run, jump, tumble, dance, wriggle, poke each other, seize and throw, into play and work that shall be healthy for mind and body, and to direct the force that makes children play with utensils, toys and the like toward the arts and industries that have most educative value. Even where the action and manipulation are of no value in themselves they may be desirable as means to intellectual or moral ends. We work against nature when we try to keep young children still. To learn by doing something is to learn with the full help of instinct. And we all know that it is for idle hands that Satan finds mischief.

[1] So called constructiveness and destructiveness are simply two extreme varieties of the instinct of manipulation.

Instincts and Capacities 27

Until recently the schools left to home and industrial life the development of the instinct of physical activity and sought to repress it in favor of purely mental activity; but with the broadening of the scope of the schools the direction of motor as well as mental habits has been accepted as an aim of systematic education, and with our present insight into the strength of the active tendencies in young children every wise teacher will adopt such methods as to make them allies rather than opponents.

Collecting.—The collecting instinct is instructive as a sample of the neglect of useful natural forces by teachers. Probably not one out of ten teachers of geography enlists this instinct in her service, though it is one of the taproots of interest in natural science. I venture the opinion that the efficiency of the teaching of so-called commercial geography could be increased ten per cent. simply by encouraging and systematizing the habits of collecting post-marks, stamps, pictures, samples of soils, agricultural and industrial products and the like.

Pugnacity.—The fighting instinct offers a useful illustration of the general superiority of substitution over repression as a means of inhibiting instincts. If punishing boys for fighting would cure them of it, the instinct would be its own cure, for the fighting itself brings physical pain enough. As we all know, mere repression is here a most uneconomical preventive, whereas the substitution of orderly boxing and wrestling, football, basket-ball and the like, often succeeds admirably. You cannot push the Niagara river back into Lake Erie and keep it there but you can, by creating new channels for it, make it drive the wheels of factories in the service of man. So often with the impulses of human nature.

The Error of Neglect.—Teachers are liable to one of two errors in their attitude toward instinctive tend-

28 *The Principles of Teaching*

encies. The first is to neglect instincts both as ends and as means, to add artificial virtues to children instead of cultivating those with which nature has already endowed them and to move children to knowledge and virtue by motives that are logically plausible, in disregard of those which original nature provides in full measure. To this extreme attitude the quiet, obedient lesson learner is the ideal pupil. Physical energy, independence, sociability and pride are rather discountenanced. Talks about the value of education, the needs of later life and the school armament of rewards and punishments are relied on to furnish the energy for school tasks. The instincts of action, curiosity and collecting, of emulation and achievement and mastery, and all the instinctive interests, are looked down upon as too childish motives or, more frequently, disregarded because of ignorance of their power.

To remind oneself that two of the noblest qualities of human nature, courage and maternal affection, are both pure instincts, should be a sufficient warning against despising natural tendencies. As for the childishness of motives based on instincts, in teaching children childish motives are just what must be used. And that these instinctive tendencies furnish the strongest of motives is the plain lesson of school experience.

The Error of Misuse.—The other error is to assume that nature is always right,—that what a child tends naturally to do, that is the thing he should be taught to do,—and to follow instinct regardless of where it leads. But the aims of education require us to lead nature oftener than to follow it; instincts are excellent servants but very dangerous masters. Natural tendencies are sometimes ends in themselves, often most useful means, and always forces that must be taken into account, but to

Instincts and Capacities 29

make them the sole guide of education will be a return to savagery.

The right attitude has been described in the first pages of this chapter. It may be summarized in these two quotations:—

"Respect then, I beg you, always, the original reactions, even when you are seeking to overcome their connection with certain objects and to supplant them with others that you wish to make the rule." (W. James, *Talks to Teachers*, p. 62) [1]

"Hence the transparent infatuation of the cheap advice, 'Trust to your children's instincts.' By all means let us study their instincts, and watch them, and tend them. In them, as we have asserted, lie our opportunities. Let us *not* trust them. For this is to forget that the only kind of instinct that is really to be trusted is that educated instinct we call a virtue." (J. MacCunn, *The Making of Character*, p. 29) [2]

§ 10. *Capacities*

The fundamental capacities of human nature are those of:—

Impression, the capacities for sensitivity of the different sense organs.

Expression, the capacities for arousing movement of the different motor organs.

Connection, the capacity to form habits.

Selection, the capacity to maintain and strengthen one mental process in preference to others.

Analysis, the capacity to break up a fact into elements, to think of and react to parts and aspects.

As manifested in actual human life, these fundamental capacities turn into many varieties of special capacities due (1) to the kind of stimulus sensed or the kind of mental fact connected or selected or analyzed (*e. g.,*

30   *The Principles of Teaching*

verbal memory, mathematical reasoning, color vision) and (2) to the mixture of capacity with interest (*e. g.,* honesty, executive ability, self-restraint). Moreover, our common words denoting capacities often refer to complexes of different capacities which together produce some important practical result (*e. g.,* leadership, scholarship, business ability).

The following are some of these concrete special capacities with which school education is particularly concerned:—[1]

The management of things.
The management of men.
The management of concrete ideas.
The management of abstract ideas and symbols.
Self-control.
Energy.
Precision.
Thoroughness.
Originality.
Cooperation.
Leadership.
Self-denial.
Self-reliance.
Refinement.
Sympathy.

The Error of Over-Emphasis.—As usually taught, the studies of the school,—reading, writing, arithmetic, oral and written composition, grammar, appreciation of the content of literature and knowledge of the facts of its history, geography, elementary science, history, alge-

[1] The capacities concerned with sensation and movement are highly important in school life, but the principles of teaching which concern them have been sufficiently emphasized in Chapter II. The very special capacities involved in the special school subjects are not mentioned because the intelligent student of teaching will rarely neglect them and because they would make too long a list.

Instincts and Capacities

bra, geometry and trigonometry, foreign languages and the special sciences,—give opportunity for the exercise of only the capacity for the management of *ideas*. Manual training and experimental work in science add certain opportunities for the management of things, but the management of men is given little or no scope in the traditional school. The school program and the teacher's methods are in fact both likely to be unfair to the boy or girl gifted in the control of tools and materials and in power to get on with and make use of other people.

Moreover one special part of the capacity to deal with ideas, namely, the capacity for thinking with abstractions and symbols, is given greater opportunity than other parts. The mathematics and grammar of the elementary school, and the mathematics and languages of the secondary school are easy and interesting in proportion as one has the ability to think with general and abstract terms and with their symbols. But school is often an uncomfortable, and perhaps an unprofitable, place for the concrete thinker, for the girl who can write poetry but can't parse, or the boy who can tell a good bargain but can't state the principle for solving problems in profit and loss. The school is the paradise for the abstract thinker, for the boy or girl who is able to think with fives and sixes, x's and y's, parallels and perpendiculars, H_2O's and NaCl's, latitude and longitude, conditions contrary to fact and clauses of purpose. The teacher is usually one who has himself been successful at this sort of thinking and so is more in sympathy with it. He may even thoughtlessly sneer at the mental ability of those who lack it. 'Your son will make a first-rate mechanic or grocer, but he isn't fit for high school,' said such a one. The proper retort would have been, 'Your school, then, is first-rate for one kind of a boy, but it isn't fit for the majority.'

32 *The Principles of Teaching*

It is true that abstract thought is the capacity which most clearly distinguishes the human from the brute intellect and is the most productive of general progress in civilization, and that every science and art requires more and more abstract and symbolic thinking in proportion as it advances. It is also true that this capacity is likely to stay dormant without systematic education, whereas the ordinary exigencies of life may sufficiently develop the capacity to deal with concrete facts. Still the school is for all, not for the few who have this capacity in large measure; and the school system which aims to serve the greatest good of the greatest number will establish curricula fitted to the concrete thinker and constructor. The wise teacher will also find ways to utilize and develop these capacities, no matter what the curriculum may be.

The Error of Neglect.—School life is likely to neglect also the capacities of originality, self-reliance, cooperation and leadership. Originality is rare and the teacher, in choosing methods well adapted to the majority, is likely to discourage it. Self-reliance is closely allied to contradiction and non-conformity to rules and directions, and the inconvenience of the latter to the teacher may make him over-favorable to a weak docility. The constant study of set lessons in text-books of the usual type aggravates this defect. Cooperation and leadership are common for purposes of mischief in school and play outside, but the traditional ideals of the class—as a company whose sole officer is the teacher, as a peasantry under a czar, or as a set of willing followers of a beloved leader—have led to the waste of opportunity for the cultivation of these important capacities.

Individual Differences.—Individuals differ in the strength of different capacities even more than in the

Instincts and Capacities

strength of different instincts. Man is a rational animal, but men vary from the stupidity of the idiot to the intellect of an Aristotle. The differences which are so obvious in the case of musical ability, verbal memory or leadership, exist in all capacities. Nature gives each a certain capital; education must learn what it is and make the most out of it. Exactly the same results must not be expected from any two children in a class. Some children will succeed with a study no matter how poor the teaching, and some children, no matter how good the teaching, will fail. The presence of capacities gives the possibilities of instruction and their amount sets limits to what instruction can achieve.

These individual differences are further complicated by the specialization of capacities. The boy who differs from his fellows by a surplus of the capacity to reason about numbers may show a deficit in the capacity to reason about grammatical forms. The specially good observer of birds may be an inferior observer of the spelling of words. Nature's endowment to an individual is in the form of scores of special gifts, some of which may exist in large measure, others in small. The teacher does not teach bright, mediocre and dull pupils, but a group of individuals each of whom possesses varying degrees of ability in different subjects and in different aspects of the same subject. There is, it is true, a general and fairly high correlation between many capacities, so that excellence in any one is somewhat prophetic of excellence in many others. But it is only somewhat; excellence in one is rarely prophetic of equal excellence in others. Only rarely is a pupil found who is at the top in everything; only rarely must a teacher endure a pupil who is proficient at nothing.

It is then unscientific and unjust for a teacher to

34 *The Principles of Teaching*

neglect a pupil because of lack of capacity in, say, the beginning reading and writing of the primary classes. In more than nine cases out of ten there is something worthy of learning which the pupil can learn well. To prescribe the same studies for all is at best a necessary evil. To make promotion depend upon any one study is to retard the progress of many pupils of high average capacity.

SUMMARY

What anyone becomes by education depends upon what he is by nature. Teaching is the utilization of natural tendencies for ideal ends. The first condition of a pupil's responses is the fund of instincts and capacities given by nature; the first step in teaching is to consider and allow for them. Good teaching discourages no worthy instinct or capacity; selects and strengthens the good by giving them exercise and rewarding them with satisfaction; eliminates or weakens the bad by disuse, substitution, and, but less often, by repression; economizes effort by not teaching prematurely what will come soon enough as a delayed tendency, and by not trying to eliminate what will pass away by itself. Good teaching so arranges the work of the school that a wide range of capacities may be utilized, and that instinctive activities and interests may make for intellectual and moral progress. Good teaching expects and adapts itself to wide individual differences in original nature.

§ 11. *Exercises*

1. Which of the following tendencies does school-life usually develop overmuch? Which does it too often neglect?

Instincts and Capacities 35

Aesthetic appreciation.   Envy.
Constructiveness.   Imitation.
Cooperativeness.   Memory.
Courage.   Rivalry.
Display.   Self-reliance.

2. Are the present arrangements of reading and writing in the curriculum most likely to err from relying on delayed instincts too soon or from appealing to transitory instincts too late?

3. How would you explain the fact that of a group of people who were asked what they enjoyed most as children in school a large percentage replied, 'Distributing pencils,' 'Going on errands,' and the like?

4. What instincts would be likely to remain dormant in a girl who never had younger children to care for? In a boy who was brought up in isolation from other boys?

5. Give an illustration of either ingenious use or wise direction of each of the following instincts and capacities:—

The instinct of manipulation.
"   "   " love of out-door life.
"   "   " affection.
"   "   " ownership.
The dramatic or personating tendency.
The capacity for rote memorizing.
"   "   " concrete learning.
"   "   " drawing.
"   "   " productive imagination.
"   "   " observation.
"   "   " leadership.

6. Name two or more channels into which the energy of the hunting instinct may be profitably turned.

7. Name five or six of the impulses which cause truancy. Which of these are due to instinctive tendencies?

36   *The Principles of Teaching*

8. How might the migratory instinct,—the tendency to roam and explore,—be made a positive help to school work?

9. Name an instinct of special help in nature-study.

10. Name an instinct of special help in manual training.

11. What is the effect on instinctive curiosity of attracting a child's attention by such questions as 'What do you suppose I'm going to do now?' followed by doing nothing new or specially attractive?

12. Which would you rather be, the child who asks such questions as 'Where were all the rocks before they were in the dirt?' and 'What does the rain do when it isn't raining?' or the teacher who makes fun of him for doing so? Why?

13. Give illustrations of children's questions that show silliness and support Bain's statement that, 'Much of the curiosity of children......is a spurious article. Frequently it is a mere display of egotism, the delight in giving trouble, in being pandered to and served. Questions are put, not for the desire of rational information, but from the love of excitement.' [3]

14. Give illustrations of children's questions that show the opposite.

15. Illustrate the employment of the instinct of general physical activity (a) in the service of geography; (b) in the service of history.

16. To get rid of envy, jealousy, cheating, etc., due to rivalry for marks, one teacher abolished the marking system altogether, another divided the class into two groups and kept only the scores of the two groups; a third teacher made a speech about the wickedness of envy and adopted rigid rules against cheating. Which do you

Instincts and Capacities 37

think had the best permanent effect on the tendency to personal rivalry? What names would you give to the three methods?

17. Name two capacities which the usual college preparatory course in the high school emphasizes. Two which it neglects.

18. From the point of view of instincts and capacities what would be the advantage of partial self-support as a feature of the education of boys from sixteen to twenty-two?

19. Supply appropriate words in the following: The most frequent faults of teaching with respect to intellectual capacities have been:— To appeal to——instead of to comprehension; to imitation instead of to——.

20. What capacities are especially involved in learning geometry? In learning science?

21. Compare physical with commercial geography with respect to the instincts and capacities to which they appeal.

22. Compare similarly the history of changes in government, the history of wars and the history of changes in social and industrial life.

23. Compare similarly the computation work of arithmetic with the work with concrete problems.

24. Name three games which give good opportunities for training in cooperation. Three which give little or none.

25. Which capacity develops earliest in life, musical capacity, literary ability or business ability?

26. State two questions about instincts and capacities which a teacher might properly investigate in the case of her class.

27. What are some questions about instincts and capacities not answered by this chapter the answers to which would interest you?

38 *The Principles of Teaching*

28. Explain or illustrate each of the following quotations :—

'The destructive tendency is probably only a modified form of the constructive.' [4]

'Education is the revealer of inequalities for which it is not responsible.' [5]

'In man, even within the domain of one and the same instinct, there is a possibility of widely different developments.' [6]

'Education ought then to be both an excitant and a restraint.' [7]

29. Which of the following statements are true? Which are false? Which are partly true and partly false? Defend your opinion in each case.

'The irrepressible life in children must be used as the chief motive-power in education.' [8]

'Men at their birth are by nature radically good.' [9]

A sinful nature has given each of our children more than seven times seven devils.

'Nothing can be more unwise than to tell a child he *must never* fight.' [10]

The child seeks 'decidedly and surely that which is in itself best; and, moreover, in a form wholly adapted to his condition.' [11]

Knowledge is to be considered as the food of the mind.

Knowledge is to be considered as a gymnasium for the mind.

'Most children enter school for the first time with minds athirst for knowledge.' [12]

'It behooves us to study nature's plan, and seek rather to aid than to thwart it. For nature must be right; there is no higher criterion.' [13]

'These instincts, then, which every child has, although

Instincts and Capacities 39

in varying form, and vigor, must be turned into worthy grooves. Not suppression, but a generous control!' [14]

§ 12. *Self-Activity*

The last four sections should have made it evident that the result of educational endeavor depends as truly upon the nature of the individual taught as upon the nature of the tuition given him. The activity from without in the shape of the words and acts of teachers, the lessons in books and the like, cooperates with the activity from within in the shape of the instincts, capacities and individual qualities of the pupils. In the last analysis what the scholars do, not what the teacher does, educates them; not what we give, but what they get, counts; only through their self-activity are they directly changed.

Education should be considered not as a moulding of perfectly plastic substances, nor as a filling of empty minds, nor as a creation of powers; but rather as the provision of opportunity for healthy bodily and mental life, of stimuli to call forth desirable activities in thought, feeling and movement, and of means for their wise direction, for the elimination of their failures and futilities, and for the selection of their useful forms.

This general point of view may be called the doctrine of self-activity. It may be stated briefly as follows: Nothing really counts except as it influences the pupil's own responses; to encourage healthy life, to stimulate to mental activity and to select the best of such activities is the teacher's work.

That the teacher must educate pupils by means of their own activities does not, however, mean that what a pupil does of his own accord is right. The teacher must constantly stimulate certain acts and prevent others;

40   *The Principles of Teaching*

must perpetuate some and eliminate others. Nor does self-activity include only such obviously active responses as the unaided discovery of facts, the invention of processes, the undirected working out of arguments. To learn by mere imitation and to commit to memory are activities as true, though not so pronounced, as original discovery. They have their place, though not so high a place, in education.

Least of all should anyone confuse self-activity with bodily activity, or take responses to mean only gross physical movements. The child who sits quietly absorbed in solving a problem is more active and more truly active than his neighbor in the next seat who is jumping up and down with glee at getting the answer. The activity of thought indeed often involves the cessation of many bodily actions.

Finally, activity may as well result in the inhibition as in the production of ideas and feelings and movements. A fifth grade school-room in which children sit quietly reading or move about in a business-like way may represent more real activity than a room in which the children are waving their hands, incessantly making comments and asking questions. The first room may, it is true, represent mere repression and absence of interest and work; but it may represent interest, thought and work *plus the inhibition of aimless expressions thereof.* It must not be forgotten that *not* to think the foolish, irrelevant thought is the essential of reasoning; that *not* to follow the wrong impulse is the essential of character; that *not* to make the aimless and crude movement is the essential of skill. Success is in great measure not making failures. What a man does depends upon what impulses are neglected or overcome. We are what we are by reason of what we are not,—what we do not per-

Instincts and Capacities 41

mit ourselves to become. Activity is inhibitory as well as impulsive.

Under the topic, *Self-Activity,* books on education often treat of the value of experiment and inference by pupils in comparison with information-giving by the teacher, of so-called developing methods in comparison with the study of conclusions as stated outright, and of reasoning in comparison with learning by rote. These and other similar matters are, however, better studied in connection with the special topic, *Reasoning,* in Chapter X.

SUMMARY

The nature of the pupil as well as the nature of the stimulus decides his response. To arouse, direct and select from his responses is the work of the teacher. Responses of perception, absorption, memory, imitation and the like are useful, though not so worthy as responses of reflection, reasoning or invention. Activities of neglect, inhibition and guidance are even more important than activities of impulsion.

For Further Reading

W. James, *Talks to Teachers on Psychology,* Chapters III-VII inclusive.

E. A. Kirkpatrick, *Fundamentals of Child Study,* Chapters III-X inclusive, XII and XIV.

CHAPTER IV

APPERCEPTION

Preparatory, *Elements of Psychology*, §§ 35-37, 42-45, 50

§ 13. *The General Law*

The general law of association and its supplément, the law of analogy or assimilation, teach that what any pupil thinks or feels or does on any occasion depends upon what he has thought and felt and done in the past and upon the present 'set' or tendency of his mind. He will respond to any stimulus in the way that he has responded to it or to some stimulus like it with resulting satisfaction. A mind's past experience and present content determine its responses. Just as education must at the start build on instincts and native capacities, so at each future step it must build on previous experience and pay heed to present conditions. If the knowledge or power needed as a preparation for the task in hand is lacking, the teacher's first duty is to secure it. This is the law of apperception.

Except in so far as unlearned tendencies of themselves provide proper responses, every act of teaching is subject to this law. To observe an object aright, the student must know certain facts about it and about what he is to look for; to attend to a lesson properly he needs to know its aim and to have knowledge with which it makes connection; to comprehend an argument he must have had training which impresses the pertinence of its steps; to

Apperception 43

be remembered a fact must have found a place in his system of thought and knowledge; to reach a conclusion properly he must have had the data; to acquire a certain technical skill in hand work he must have reached the necessary point of motor development.

To proceed from the known to the related unknown, from rough preliminary knowledge to detailed and adequate knowledge, from simple facts to complex facts depending on them, to teach one thing at a time,—are rules each referring to one aspect of the general law of apperception. As nine-tenths of human life and learning illustrates the general law of association, so nine-tenths of teaching illustrates the use or abuse of the law of apperception. The teaching of reading depends largely upon knowledge of spoken language and of common things and events; the teaching of algebra relies upon knowledge of arithmetic; the teaching of multiplication, upon knowledge of addition; the teaching of the geography of North America, upon experience of the physical features of the neighborhood; a child's attitude toward his teacher depends upon his experience with previous teachers; appreciation of literature requires knowledge of the meanings of words. The past is everywhere the key to the present.

§ 14. Detailed Applications: Exercises

The student should have gained a thorough knowledge of the meaning and scope of apperception in the learner (that is, of the laws of association and analogy or assimilation) from the study of dynamic psychology.[1] To give full realization of apperception as a principle of

---

[1] The references under 'Preparatory' will provide this knowledge and prepare the student for the exercises.

44   *The Principles of Teaching*

teaching and to form the habit of judging the value of every stimulus, not by what it is in itself, but by what it will be to the pupil or class, is the aim of the exercises that follow.

1.   How would a ten year old boy brought up in an American city probably interpret 'He gave him two guineas'?

2.   How does your own previous experience or so-called 'apperceptive mass' influence your answer?

3.   Give an illustration from school life of a mistake due to the lack of proper previous experience.

4.   Give one due to the presence of unsuitable present content.

5.   A teacher in New York City took a class to Riverside Park (situated along the Hudson River) showed them the river, called attention to its size and then said, 'Now tell us the name of this great river.' 'The Amazon,' was the prompt reply! What would you suggest as a possible explanation? What precautions would it be wise for that teacher to take on another similar excursion?

6.   It is hard to realize the lack of knowledge of pupils. Can the reader believe, for example, that a bright girl, a graduate of the grammar school, was greatly surprised to see apples growing on trees or that an intelligent eight-year-old boy in a city of over twenty thousand inhabitants was doubtful as to whether some coins given to him were pennies or nickels? Give two or three similar instances.

Experiment 2.   Write without help answers to the following questions:—

What is the price of a ton of good hay?

How many members has the House of Commons?

Where is the pituitary body?

Apperception 45

How big is a scallop?

What is the shape of a tomato leaf?

Which way do the seeds in an apple point?

What is a dumb-waiter?

What is the opposite of 'if'?

What does this mean, 'He is going to take the L'?

What is sold in a delicatessen shop?

Compare your answers with the right ones. Should these questions be much harder for you than the following would be for a six-year-old entering school?

How long is two feet?

How many legs has a pig?

Where is your heart?

How big is a cow?

What is the shape of a pine tree?

Where does the sun rise?

What does a baker do?

What does rich mean?

What does this mean, 'He went away up the mountain'?

What grows on a farm?

Experiment 3. Arrange with some one in a country school, and also with some friend in a city school, to test one by one eight or ten children in the lowest class as follows and record their answers. Compare the two groups.

How big is a loaf of bread?

" " " a horse?

" " " a cow?

What does a teacher do?

" " a policeman do?

" " a farmer do?

Experiment 4. Have your two friends also each read to eight or ten children in the second grade of the school

46 *The Principles of Teaching*

(it will be better to take them apart one at a time, but this is not absolutely necessary) selection A, without comment and have them draw pictures to tell the story. Let the story be read twice. Compare the drawings of the two groups. State briefly how their drawings illustrate the fact of apperception. Make the same experiment with selection B.

A.

One day a fox came out of the woods near our house, and tried to catch a hen in the barn. But the hens saw him and made a great noise. Hero was in the yard, and he ran into the barn and drove the fox off. Hero did not catch him, but he barked so loud that the fox ran for his life back to the woods. He did not get one of our hens for his dinner that day. Is not Hero a good dog? [15]

B.

Carl was a little lame boy. He lived in an attic with his mother. He used to look out of the window and watch the boys at play. He could see the men and the women and the horses and wagons in the street. One day there was a little baby playing in the street when the trolley car came around the corner. She was on the track right in front of it. Carl gave a scream, for he was afraid the baby would be run over. But just then a big dog ran out into the street, took hold of the baby's dress with his teeth and carried her back to the sidewalk to her big sister.

7. How does the principle of apperception apply to teaching the spelling of compound words?

8. Make an argument of about one hundred words on the basis of the law of apperception in favor of beginning the study of geography with home geography.

9. In what respect would this law support the practice of beginning United States History with the discovery of America by Columbus and following the order of time?

10. In what respect would it support the opposite

Apperception 47

practice of beginning with an account of the nation as it now is, giving next a brief picture of national life 'when your fathers and mothers were little boys and girls,' giving next a brief picture of the nation a hundred years ago and then one of the nation in 1700, and only then passing to the early voyagers and colonists and tracing events and changes in conditions of life in chronological order?

11. What is the previous experience necessary before the definition of a pronoun can be taught properly?

12. What argument for stating clearly the aim of a lesson do you draw from the principle of apperception?

13. What argument for the use of reviews?

14. Considering a review lesson from the point of view of apperception alone, which facts should be reviewed?

15. How does the fact of apperception help to account for the relatively inferior teaching of substitute teachers?

16. What is the experience or apperceptive basis necessary for the comprehension of the meaning of such words of relationship as *this, which, nevertheless* and *its?*

17. Of the two factors which determine a pupil's response, (a) his previous experience of the stimulus and of other stimuli like it and (b) the temporary 'set' of his mind, which has the greater influence?

18. Which is influenced by stating the aim of a lesson?

19. Why is it often not a loss of time to ask questions which every member of the class is able to answer?

20. Give two or more illustrations of gross neglect of the mental content of a pupil such as the following: " 'Will you please tell me why I carry one for every ten,' said little Laura to her instructor. 'Yes, my dear,' said

48   *The Principles of Teaching*

she kindly. 'It is because numbers increase from left to right in a decimal ratio.' "[1]

In the case of teaching about the physical world as in physical geography, physics, chemistry, botany, zoology, human physiology and the like, the first hand observation of the objects themselves is the experience necessary to adequate knowledge of their structure, properties, relations and actions. Without such an apperceptive basis, there is a high probability that the knowledge gained will not connect with reality or modify responses to actual situations of life and there is some danger of its being exclusively verbal.

21. Apply this same principle to the question of the use of 'sources' in history.

22. How then would you teach the fact of the transportation of soil by water?

23. Apply the principle of the above paragraph to the teaching of the tables of weights, measures and foreign money.

24. What would be advisable as preparatory lessons before giving a book-lesson on the constitution of water? By what would you replace the book-lesson if you were unfettered by practical limitations?

25. What would be your first steps in teaching a class the function of the cotyledons of the bean?

26. In teaching the structure and action of the human heart?

27. Name five cases in which first hand acquaintance with the things themselves is out of question?

28. Name five cases such as the study of bacteria in the high school where the practical difficulties of giving direct acquaintance with the object to be studied outweigh the advantages.

[1] The author regrets that he is unable to give the source of this charming illustration of the frying pan and fire in teaching.

Apperception 49

29. Illustrate the profitable use of a school museum; of school excursions; of demonstrations of experiments in elementary science; of a school garden.

In emphasizing the importance of paying heed to the past experience and present frame of mind of a pupil, one is likely to forget that we pay heed to them only in order to add to them. Good teaching will fit its stimuli to the pupil's knowledge, but only in order to increase it; good teaching will work on his actual present tendency, but only to improve it. In the familiar recommendation, *To proceed to the unknown* is as important as *from the*

A.

CLASS WORK.	SEAT WORK.
Talk about things of which the pupils can see two of a kind, — as two hands, two boys, etc.	Make two lines on your slates, thus:
Let the pupils name objects of which they see two of a kind.	Make two lines, thus:
EXAMPLES: " I see two boys.; I have two feet; here are two sticks."	
"How many sticks have I here?" ("One.")	Make two dots, ● ●
"How many in my other hand?" ("One.")	Make two rings, O O
"Now how many?" [Putting them together.] ("Two.")	Make two stars, ✳ ✳
"Then one stick and one stick are how many?"	Put two dots together like these ⁝, or these ●, or these ●.
"One and one are how many?"	Put two stars together in the same way.
Illustrate in the same way with balls, pencils, nails, and other objects.	Put two rings together in the same way.
"I strike the bell once; I strike it once again. How many times did I strike it?" [16]	Make two lines cross each other, thus:
	Make two lines meet each other, thus:

4

50　　*The Principles of Teaching*

known. To simply review the known, to elaborate at length what pupils have long been familiar with, is a more harmful violation of the principle of apperception than to overwhelm them with facts which they cannot assimilate. Incomprehensibility is no worse than monotonous repetition. Indigestion is not so bad as starvation.

30. What do you think of giving as the first work in arithmetic fourteen pages of such drill on the number 2 as is exemplified in A.?

31. Collect from text-books four or more illustrations of the sort of violation of the principle of apperception mentioned in the paragraph preceding Question 30. State wherein each one violates the principle.

For Further Reading

W. James, *Talks to Teachers on Psychology,* Chapter XIV.

J. Adams, *Herbartian Psychology Applied to Education,* Chapter III.

C. A. McMurry and F. M. McMurry, *The Method of the Recitation,* Chapter VI.

CHAPTER V

INTERESTS

§ 15. *The Meaning of Interests*

When any situation arouses attention, that is, leads the mind to busy itself with the thing or idea or feeling, it is called interesting. The tendency to devote one's thought and action to a fact is called interest in it. The feeling of arousal, of mental zest, of being drawn to the fact, is called the feeling of interest.

With the fact and feeling of interest education is concerned in two ways: First, it must be the aim of education to encourage and create desirable and to discourage and destroy undesirable interests. From this point of view interests are an end. Second, we depend upon interests to furnish the motives for the acquisition of knowledge and for the formation of right habits of thought and action. From this second point of view interests are a means. Thus the interest in nature, in our physical surroundings and in animals and plants, the interest in bodily health and vigor, and the interest in truth, are ends for which education strives. Thus the interest in bodily movement and the interest in ownership are means by which children are led to gain skill and effectiveness in constructive work, drawing, cooking and the like.

This distinction is important, for a majority of the errors made in teaching with respect to interests are due to confusing means and ends.

52 The Principles of Teaching

Interests may be native or acquired. Many human instincts are unlearned tendencies not to do something, but to take attitudes of interest or aversion. There are, that is, instinctive interests or instincts of interest. Many human habits are habits not of out and out thought or action, but of attitude, of interest and aversion. In general, then, the educational principles based on the psychology of instincts and habits are applicable to interests as well.

§ 16. *Interests as Ends*

The Control of Interests.—Not all natural interests are desirable. To destroy the interest in coarse excitement is as necessary a work as to develop the interest in good reading. As with all instincts and habits, nature's tendencies are not safe guides to education's ideals. The destruction may be, as with all instincts, by giving the undesirable interest no chance for exercise, by forming the habit of meeting in some other way the situation concerned, (*i. e.,* by substitution or redirection), and by actual repression by discomfort. Desirable interests are perpetuated, of course, by furnishing the stimuli that arouse them and by rewarding them with satisfaction. The capital with which an individual starts is the native interests, the instincts of interest in movement, novelty, color, action, living animals, excitement, rhythm, the opposite sex and the like. The problem is to select for continuance the good and to graft the interest to be acquired upon some interest already present, or rather to develop out of some interest already present the one which we seek. Thus from the interest in constructing a boat may be developed an interest in making accurate measurements; from the interest in action and excitement

Interests 53

a wise school system gradually obtains an interest in history and literature.

Three Causes of Interest.—Much assistance is given to the teacher in this process of refining and redirecting interests by three facts. The first is the general law of association that whatever tendency brings satisfaction will be perpetuated and strengthened. Whenever an interest is made to profit a pupil, it will be preserved. Connect any response with an original or acquired satisfier and it will satisfy. The hardest sort of bodily labor becomes interesting when it gives a boy a place on the football team or connects with the excitement and achievement of hunting big game. The second is the force of imitation. What the community cares about will interest each new member; the teacher who is interested in a subject will infect her class. The third is the fact that knowledge breeds interest, that, with certain exceptions, the power to handle a subject produces in the long run an interest in it, uninteresting as it may have been at the start. As soon as the high-school pupil can really read German, he is likely to gain an interest in it.

Errors in Teaching.—In cultivating interests the chief danger is in mistaking one for another and so getting the wrong one. The boy may be thought to play football because of an interest in bodily perfection and athletic sport when his real motive is the interest in seeing his name in the paper, being applauded by large audiences, and being admired and envied by his fellows. The girl may be thought to possess a real interest in knowledge when her efforts are really only to beat Mary who failed to graduate.

The chief defect of school instruction with respect to the acquisition of interests is that, as a consequence, they are not permanent. Interests are present under the

54 *The Principles of Teaching*

stimuli of school life which die out soon after it is completed. As children we learn, but as adults we too often lose our love for learning: the higher feelings are nourished in the protected surroundings of the college, but do not long survive the transfer to the rougher outside world and competition with the interests in money, power and position.

§ 17. *Interests as Means*

All Work Implies Interest.—To a normal boy or girl physical or mental work without interest is an impossibility. When one does the most uninteresting work he still does it from interest,—interest in the avoidance of punishment, in maintaining his standing in class or in preserving his self-respect. Interest of some sort there must be.

The problem of interest in teaching is not whether children shall learn with interest or without it; they never learn without it; but what kind of interest it shall be; from what the interest shall be derived.[1] There need be no quarrel between those who say all work should be made interesting and those who say all proper work should be done whether it is interesting or not. For both statements are true. The actual difference of opinion is about whether we should in large measure derive interests in school work from the common instinctive interests in play, action, novelty, emulation and the like, or should derive them from the abstract and rare interests in duty and knowledge. The latter interests are the higher and if they are present it is well to appeal to them. But in

---

[1] When an individual is attracted by the intrinsic qualities of the work his interest may be called *immediate* or *intrinsic;* when the work does not interest him in and of itself but only by its consequences or connections, the interest is called *derived.*

Interests 55

actual school work the choice is commonly not between the common instinctive interests and these higher ones,— not between, for instance, curiosity and love of pure truth,—but between one common interest and another, between, for instance, curiosity and fear of punishment.

Practical Precepts.—The practical rules are simple: Having decided what an individual or a class ought to learn, arouse as much interest in it as is needed; get interest, but derive it from the best interest available. Other things being equal, get interest that is steady and self-sustaining rather than interest that flags repeatedly and has to be constantly reinforced by thoughts of duty, punishment or the like. Get the right things done at any cost,—but get them done with as little inhibition and strain as possible. Other things being equal, work with and not against instinctive interests.

There is in reality not so much conflict between what children ought to learn and what is interesting to them as we often imagine. It is true that their interests in crude excitement, novel sensations, silly plays and the like work against their true progress, but it is also true that *our* failure to enter into the spirit of child-life, our neglect of their real needs, the unfitness of many of our methods to employ and interpret their intellectual life work equally against their true progress. To choose as the subject matter of instruction facts which are as remote from any real demands of a child's intellect as the geometry of a space of n dimensions is from any real demands of our own and then to seek to conjure up an interest in them is a poor solution of the problem of interest. One factor that should decide what children ought to learn and do is adaptation to the intellectual and practical needs which the children can then and there appreciate; and this factor is also a chief determinant of their interests,

56 *The Principles of Teaching*

"And so has come up the modern theory and practice of the 'interesting,' in the false sense of that term. The material is still left; so far as its own characteristics are concerned, just material externally selected and formulated. It is still just so much geography and arithmetic and grammar study; not so much potentiality of child-experience with regard to language, earth, and numbered and measured reality. Hence the difficulty of bringing the mind to bear upon it; hence its repulsiveness; the tendency for attention to wander; for other acts and images to crowd in and expel the lesson. The legitimate way out is to transform the material; to psychologize it—that is, once more, to take it and to develop it within the range and scope of the child's life. But it is easier and simpler to leave it as it is, and then by trick of method to *arouse* interest, to *make* it *interesting;* to cover it with sugar-coating; to conceal its barrenness by intermediate and unrelated material; and finally, as it were, to get the child to swallow and digest the unpalatable morsel while he is enjoying tasting something quite different. But alas for the analogy! Mental assimilation is a matter of consciousness; and if the attention has not been playing upon the actual material, that has not been apprehended, nor worked into faculty." (J. Dewey, *The Child and the Curriculum,* p. 38.) [17]

False Views of Interest.—It is a common error to confuse the interesting with the easy and to argue that the doctrine of interest is false because it is wrong to make everything easy. This is an error because in fact the most difficult things may be very interesting and the easiest things very dull. Walking, scribbling and nodding are not more interesting than running, drawing pictures and making up faces. Indeed difficulty is of itself rather interesting than otherwise.

The real facts are that work at which one utterly fails, with which one makes no headway, is commonly uninteresting, that the same thing becomes easier to an individual when attacked with interest, and that to any

Interests 57

individual those lines of work for which he possesses capacity are commonly interesting.

Two things may be meant when a study or lesson is called hard; (1) that it is generally so regarded and (2) that the individual doing it finds it hard. It would be a cowardly principle of teaching to omit work merely because it was hard in the first sense. But it would equally be the height of folly to despise an individual's work merely because *he* found it easy. The obvious course is to face bravely the tasks that are commonly esteemed hard and then do everything that can properly be done to make them as easy as may be.

A second common error is to confuse the feeling of interest with pleasure and to argue that we cannot make school work interesting because some necessary features of it simply are not pleasurable. It is of course true that many things must be done by a school pupil which produce no pleasure, but they may nevertheless be done with interest. A tug of war and putting up the heavy dumb-bell the fiftieth time are definitely painful, but may be very interesting.

A third common error is to over-estimate the strength of children's interests in abstract thinking such as characterizes the logical aspects of arithmetic, formal grammar, deductive geometry and the syntax of foreign languages. In high schools where the pupils represent a selection of the more capable and scholarly, the teacher may depend upon a fair amount of the interest in mental gymnastics, in thought regardless of its content. But even in high schools this interest will be slight in a majority of cases and in the grammar school it is never safe to depend on it as a motive for a class. For the majority of all minds and the great majority of untutored

58 *The Principles of Teaching*

minds demand content, mental stuff, actual color, movement, life and 'thingness' as their mental food.

There are two failures of teaching with respect to interest. The first is the failure to arouse any mental zest in a class, to lift the class out of a dull, listless, apathetic good behavior or keep them from illicit interests in grinning at each other, playing tricks, chewing candy and the like. This we all recognize as failure. The second type succeeds in getting interest, but the interest is in the wrong thing. Many a class sit entranced as the teacher shows them pictures—they are thoroughly interested and attentive—but they have no interest whatever in the principle or fact which the pictures are to illustrate. A lecturer can always get interest by telling funny stories, but again and again he will find that the real content of his lecture has been entirely neglected. Too often the picture, the story, the specimen or the experiment removes as much interest from the lesson itself by distracting the pupil as it adds by its concreteness, life and action. It is never enough to keep a class interested. They must be interested in the right thing.

SUMMARY

Some interests are ends; all interests may under proper circumstances be used as means.

Good teaching perpetuates desirable instinctive interests, using the same methods as in the case of instincts, and creates interests in facts that are not originally attractive by connecting them with facts that are. Its goal is interests in these facts for their own sake.

Good teaching decides what is to be learned by an appeal not to interest, but to the general aim of education. Having so decided, it secures interest—the most, the best and the steadiest possible. Other things being equal it uses instinctive rather than artificial interests

Interests 59

and common rather than rare interests. It is ever on the watch against mistaking one interest for another.

§ 18. *Exercises*

1. Name two or three interests which are ends in education.

2. Name two or three interests which are only means.

3. Illustrate the development of the interest in other people (the so-called social instinct) as an end.

4. Illustrate its use as a means in teaching history. In teaching German.

5. (a) Of the interests mentioned below name five that are largely instinctive. (b) Two that are largely acquired. (c) Two that are long delayed. (d) Three that appear early in life and also stay late. (e) Three that education should commonly weaken. (f) The two that are commonest. (g) The two that are rarest. (h) Three that are risky as motives in school.

In excitement.
In getting money.
In mechanical contrivances.
In moving rather than still things.
In the other sex.
In romance.
In adventure.
In living animals.
In one's personal affairs.
In society.
In novelty.
In music.
In rhythm.
In ownership.

60   *The Principles of Teaching*

In abstract thinking.
In adornment.
In the stock exchange.
In philosophy.

6. What sentence in the text is illustrated by the following? To develop good interests in art one should surround young children with pictures that not only are of artistic merit, but also possess the qualities of action, color or story-telling and which deal with subjects which children care about.

7. How would you develop an interest in chemistry out of an interest in cooking?

8. What common interests of boyhood might be used as a starting point for or reinforcement of the interest in chemistry?

9. Business men complain that the graduates of the schools can rarely write an effective letter. Pupils complain that composition is dry and uninteresting work. The same pupils who show little interest in school tasks often become absorbed in the serious study of some trade or profession as soon as they have decided to make it their occupation in life. Putting the three facts just mentioned together and recalling the first of the three aids to teachers in redirecting interests, arrange a plan for securing interest in composition writing in the high school.

10. What is the danger in relying exclusively on artificial motives, external rewards and punishments, trusting that when sufficient knowledge has been gained an interest in the subject itself will develop?

11. What interest is added to a subject for a student when he chooses it himself instead of being compelled to take it?

12. How would you cure a boy of an interest in

Interests 61

cheap blood-and-thunder stories? Of an interest in display, in 'showing-off'?

13. What do you think makes the stories of *Cinderella*, of *Little Red Riding Hood* and of *The Three Bears* so interesting to small children?

14. How would you explain the following case of marked interest in what most people would call an uninteresting thing? 'I have seen a roomful of college students suddenly become perfectly still, to look at their professor of physics tie a piece of string around a stick which he was going to use in an experiment, but immediately grow restless when he began to explain the experiment.' [18]

15. The interests in the concrete and in action can often be made of service in the most abstract subjects; *e. g.*, paper-folding is of help in learning geometry. Illustrate the same general fact in the case of learning the forms of the letters.

16. Illustrate the wise use of each of the following interests as a means to gaining knowledge or skill:—The interest in ownership. The interest in money-making. The interest in living animals.

17. Name three interests which contribute to make pupils eager to know their marks. Which of these are desirable, and which undesirable, interests?

18. What would be the advantage of repeating a test (without warning, of course) after a month and giving to each pupil as a mark the amount of gain made over his record of a month before?

19. Illustrate the wise use of the dramatic instinct in the primary school. In the high school.

20. One of the strongest of human tendencies is to resist being balked or frustrated in the execution of any impulse after one has begun to act upon it. Give cases

62 *The Principles of Teaching*

of difficulty in managing children due to failure to make allowance for this tendency.

21. How could you utilize the interest of high-school boys in inventions and mechanical contrivances?

22. How might you perhaps utilize their interest in strength and bodily symmetry as an aid in the study of Greek? In the study of physiology?

23. Name one result on school work of each of the following interests of adolescence? The interest in the other sex. The interest in self-direction, in being one's own master. The interest in religion.

24. Which of the two following lists of topics for compositions is the better adapted to secure the interest of high-school classes?

A Canoeing Trip.	The Duties of a Full-back.
How to Choose a Bicycle.	Building a Boat.
Spring House-cleaning.	The Construction of a Shot-
The Appearance of Church	gun.
on Easter Sunday.	
The Prospects of our Base-	
ball Team.	
Nursing as a Profession.	

25. Consider the characters presented to students for emulation in school courses in history and in reading-books, from the point of view of your answer to Question 24. What changes are needed to secure better adaptation to the interests of all students?

26. What interests are appealed to by a mental arithmetic recitation?

27. In what per cent. (roughly) of high-school pupils does geometry really appeal to the interest in pure reasoning?

28. Some one has said that we should study Latin to know how the Romans thought and felt. From what

Interests

63

interests does the high-school pupil usually study Latin?

29. When is it justifiable (or least objectionable) to use a bad interest as a motive for school work?

30. What was Miss Bessie's error in the teaching described in the following?

"It had seemed to Miss Bessie advisable that the 'children should know something of the world on which they live,' and for purposes of instruction she had selected a geyser and a volcano as important—not to say interesting—features of land structure. By means of a rubber ball with a hole in it, artfully concealed in a pile of sand, she had created a geyser, and with a bit of cotton soaked in alcohol and lighted she had simulated a volcano.

"We began our work with geography in ignorance of these facts. After a few lessons on hills, mountains, islands, capes, and bays, the children informed us that they 'didn't like those old things.' 'Please, won't you give us the fireworks?' asked Freddie. 'Or the squirt?' added Agnes eagerly." [19]

Experiment 5. Ask the children of a third or fourth grade class each to draw a picture of whatever they like. Examine their drawings. What is the predominant interest, in technical ability, in ornamentation, in making the drawing pretty or in expressing facts?

Experiment 6. (a) Spend a Saturday afternoon in the reading-room of a public library or Young Men's Christian Association building. Make a plan of the room, locating the different magazines. Observe and record in the case of each boy from fifteen to eighteen years of age, which magazine he looks for first and which second (in case the first choice is in use). State briefly the facts you observe and the conclusions about the interests of boys of the high-school age which you draw from them.

(b) If the above is impracticable, get some friend to ask the boys of a third or fourth year high-school class to each cross out from the list given below the names of

64 *The Principles of Teaching*

those magazines about which they know nothing and then to mark the most interesting of those left (1) and the next most interesting (2).

McClure's Magazine.   Forest and Stream.
Outing.   The Century Magazine.
The Scientific American   Boyhood.
The Youth's Companion.   Life.

State briefly the facts and conclusions as in (a).

Experiment 7. Which of the three selections, A, B and C, is the most interesting to children in the second year of school? What accounts for its superiority?

Pick out the least interesting features of each selection. State why they lack interest.

Discuss each selection briefly (in from thirty to fifty words) from the point of view of interest.

How did you decide which was the most interesting? What would be the best way to decide?

A.
MR. LONGFELLOW

This is a picture of Mr. Longfellow.
He was the boy who lived near the sea.
He is an old gentleman in this picture.
He still loved the birds and flowers.
His heart was always kind.
He was a poet.
A poet has beautiful thoughts.
He writes them for others to read.
His thoughts make people better.
When he was a boy he went to school.
Then he went to Bowdoin College.
Bowdoin College is in Maine.
He then went across the ocean.
He spent four years in other countries.
When he came back he was a teacher in Bowdoin College.
He lived afterwards in Cambridge, Massachusetts.
He went there to teach in Harvard College. [20]

Interests 65

B.
KING TAWNY MANE

1. Here is a fable that comes to us from India. It has amused the children of that country for a great many years; and, while you are trying to find the lesson which it teaches, it may also amuse you.

2. There was once a lion whose name was Tawny Mane. He was so strong that all the other animals were afraid of him, and so he was called the king of the forest. He liked to kill every animal that came in his way, and there was no living thing in all the land that was safe from him.

3. At last, one day, all the animals met to talk about their troubles, and see if they could not find some plan to save themselves from King Tawny Mane. They talked a long time, and then agreed what to do.

4. In the evening they went together to the lion's den. King Tawny Mane had just had a full meal, and so he did not try to harm any of them. "What do you want here?" he roared.

5. This frightened them very much. Some of them ran back into the thick woods. But the bravest stood still. "Speak, and tell me what you want," said the king.

6. Then Sharp Ears, the fox, stood up and spoke. "O king," he said, "we have come to see you about a very great matter. Do you know that if you keep on as you have begun, you will soon kill all the beasts in the forest?"

7. "And what if I do?" said Tawny Mane. "Then what will become of you?" said Sharp Ears. "What kind of a king will you be when you have killed all your subjects?"

8. "But I must have something to eat," said Tawny Mane. "I must have food."

9. "Yes," said Sharp Ears, "and that is just what we have come to talk about. We have thought of a plan by which you shall have all the food you want without going out of doors to get it."

10. "That would be a good plan," said Tawny Mane. "But tell me what it is."

5

66 *The Principles of Teaching*

11. "We will give you one animal every day," said Sharp Ears. "We will draw lots, and the one upon whom the lot falls shall come to your den. You will not have to hunt at all."

12. "Good!" said the king. "We will try your plan, and see how we like it."

13. For some time after this, things were very quiet in the forest. Every morning one of the animals went down into Tawny Mane's den, and never came out again. The lion liked the new plan quite well.

14. At last the lot fell upon a little rabbit named Cotton Tail, and he was sent to make a call upon the king. He was in no hurry to go. He played along the road until after dinner time. Then, with big eyes and gentle steps, he went and stood at the lion's door.

15. King Tawny Mane was very hungry, and when he saw the rabbit he roared, "Why are you so late? Even the elephant knows better than to keep me waiting."

16. The rabbit bowed low and said, "I know I am late. But if you could only see what I have seen, you would not blame me."

17. "What have you seen?" said the lion.
"I have seen something that may have a good deal to do with your keeping this kingdom," said Cotton Tail.

18. "Tell me about it," said the lion. He was always afraid that something would happen to drive him out of his kingdom.

19. "I can not tell you," said Cotton Tail, "but if you will come with me, I will show you what I saw." Then he hopped away, and the lion followed him until they came to the mouth of an old well. At the bottom of the well there was a little water, and under the water there was nothing but soft sand.

20. "Just look in here," said Cotton Tail.
King Tawny Mane looked in. He thought he saw another lion at the bottom of the well. He showed his teeth; the other lion showed his teeth. "I am the king of the forest!" roared Tawny Mane. The other lion said nothing; but Tawny Mane thought that he roared.

21. "I will show you that I am the king," growled

Interests 67

Tawny Mane. He was so angry that he did not know what to do. He jumped into the well, only to find that there was nothing but water and soft sand at the bottom. He could not get out.

22. Then little Cotton Tail peeped down and called to the lion. "Tawny Mane," he said, "your kingdom is at an end!"

23. Little by little, Tawny Mane sank in the sand. In the evening Cotton Tail peeped down again. All was still.

24. After that, the rabbit was looked upon as a great hero of the forest. But when the other beasts wanted to make him their king, he said, "No! I am only a rabbit, and I do not want to be a king." [21]

C.

Food

We must never forget that we do not live to eat, but that we eat to live.

Our food is the flesh of beasts, birds, and fish, and the fruits of the earth.

Beef is the flesh of the ox, pork is the flesh of the pig, and mutton is the flesh of the sheep.

Apples grow on trees, and grapes grow on vines. Turnips and beets grow in the ground.

Bread and cake are made of flour. Tea is the leaf of a bush which grows in the far East. Coffee is the seed of a berry which grows on a tree.

Salt, which is put into most of our food, is got from mines, or from salt-water wells. [22]

For Further Reading

W. James, *Talks to Teachers on Psychology*, Chapter X.

J. Adams, *Herbartian Psychology Applied to Education*, Chapter X.

CHAPTER VI

INDIVIDUAL DIFFERENCES

§ 19. *Variability in General*

Common observation shows that children differ greatly in their mental make-up and psychology proves these differences to exist in the case of all mental qualities and to be of the utmost practical importance. In the physical characteristics of the sense and motor organs, in the strength of instincts and capacities, in the nature of their previous experiences and inborn and acquired interests— no two children are exactly alike and any one school class will show extensive differences. The same stimulus cannot be expected to produce exactly the same response in any two and will rarely produce anything like the same response from all.

Such variations exist throughout living nature; trees do not all grow equally fast, seeds will not all produce equal crops, one hundred horses will not be equally fast or strong; but the variations in human intellect and character are especially great in amount and complex in character.

The Nature of Mental Differences.—It is a common but absolutely false notion that in any quality or combination of qualities children can be divided into a 'normal' group all closely alike and a group of exceptional children differing widely from the normal. On the contrary, the form of distribution of mental traits is

Individual Differences

commonly continuous,—is such that people are found possessing every grade of ability from the highest to the lowest, every amount of the quality from the greatest to the least. Thus in addition people do not fall into two or three sharply defined classes, average adders, good adders and bad adders, but range as shown in the measurements given below of eighty-three seventh-grade pupils (Table I). Children are not active or inert, but vary all the way from greatest to least strength of the instinct of physical activity. They are not bright, average and dull, but are very, very bright, very bright, less bright, still less bright, about half way from the brightest to the dullest, somewhat dull, duller, very dull and very, very dull, with a practically infinite variety of grades in between.

TABLE I.

In a test in addition, all pupils being allowed the same time.

1 pupil did		3	examples	correctly
2 pupils "		4	"	"
1	" "	5	"	"
5	" "	6	"	"
2	" "	7	"	"
4	" "	8	"	"
6	" "	9	"	"
14	" "	10	"	"
8	" "	11	"	"
7	" "	12	"	"
8	" "	13	"	"
5	" "	14	"	"
5	" "	15	"	"
6	" "	16	"	"
1	" "	17	"	"
5	" "	18	"	"
1	" "	19	"	"
2	" "	20	"	"

Their Amount.—Small differences are more frequent than large ones. In the case of the addition ability

70   *The Principles of Teaching*

described above a patient reader can figure out that there are about 240 times as many differences of 1 as there are of 17, that there are 70 times as many differences of 2 or less as there are of 15 or more, and that there are about 8 times as many differences of 0 to 8 as there are of 9 to 17. And in general the form of distribution is such that between very many individuals the differences are little, that between many they are moderate and that between a few only are they very great. The exact facts in the case of the abilities of the seventh-grade pupils in addition are as shown in Table II.

TABLE II.

Of the 3403 differences between one seventh-grade pupil and another of the 83 tested in addition,

247	were differences of	0	amount
476	"	"	1	"
460	"	"	2	"
420	"	"	3	"
382	"	"	4	"
334	"	"	5	"
282	"	"	6	"
219	"	"	7	"
188	"	"	8	"
126 .	"	"	9	"
109	"	"	10	"
53	"	"	11	"
48	"	"	12	"
26	"	"	13	"
18	"	"	14	"
10	"	"	15	"
3	"	"	16	"
2	"	"	17	"

In the case of the ability in addition we notice also that the different grades of ability are by no means equally frequent, but that all the cases cluster around the abilities 10 to 13 (see Table I). This fact becomes even clearer if one pictures the frequency of each of the different grades of ability by the size of an area as in FIG. 1 and FIG. 2.

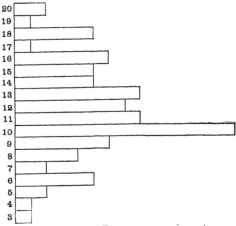

FIG. 1.

FIG. 1. The different abilities in addition are denoted on a vertical scale, 3 meaning 3 examples done correctly, 4 meaning 4 examples done correctly, and so on for 5, 6, 7, 8, etc. The number of pupils who were of each ability is denoted by the horizontal length of the column in each case, each sixth of an inch of horizontal length standing for one individual. Thus there was 1 pupil who did only 3 examples correctly, 1 who did only 4 examples, 2 who did 5, 5 who did 6 and so on. It is obvious at a glance that there are far more individuals, *i. e.* that there is a far larger surface, in the middle third of the scale than in the lower or in the upper third.

In any group of the same general class with respect to age or training, such a clustering of the cases, commonly around a medium degree of the ability, will be the case. Individuals, that is, vary about a central type, so that we can think of any single individual's ability as a plus or minus deviation from the central tendency or type of his age, sex or grade. Tables III to VIII show this in the case of the distribution of six different abilities. The facts of Tables III-VIII are presented graphically in FIGS. 3-8.

The amount of difference actually found in children

of the same age or in children in the same school grade is greater than teachers perhaps realize. The range of ability in school children[1] of the same age is such that in

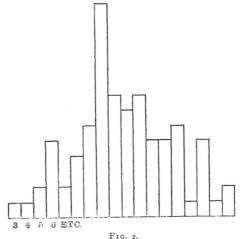

FIG. 2.

FIG. 2. This is constructed on the same general principle as FIG. 1, the difference being that in FIG. 2 the scale of ability is drawn from left to right instead of from low down to high up. Hence in this case, the *vertical* length of the columns represents the number of pupils, *i. e.*, the frequency of eachil ab ity.

a majority of capacities the most gifted child will, in comparison with the least gifted child of the same age, do over six times as much in the same time or do the same amount with less than a sixth as many errors. The samples given in Tables III, IV and VII and FIGS. 3, 4 and 7 give a concrete idea of the amount of the differences between children of the same year-age in representative capacities.

If the best speller of a class can spell correctly such

[1] These figures are true for the children whom teachers have in regular classes,—for such children as are not so far below the average as to fail to get on at all in school. If pronounced defectives were included the range of differences would be still greater.

Individual Differences

73

words as fatiguing, appreciate, delicious, guarantee, triumph and accident, the worst speller will barely spell such words as house, dollar, potato, present, severe and praise. If the weakest pupil of a class in computation can do five examples in ten minutes the best pupil will probably do at least twenty. Roughly speaking, the teacher of a class, even in a school graded as closely as is possible in large cities where two classes are provided in each building for each grade and where promotion occurs every six months, will find in the case of any kind of work some pupil who can do from two to five times as much in the same time or do the same amount from two to five times as well as some other pupil. The highest tenth of her class will in any one trait have an average ability from one and three-fourths to four times that of the lowest tenth. Even if she picks out the half of the class

TABLE III. The abilities of 11 year olds in addition.			TABLE IV. The rapidity of movement of 10 year old girls.	
Scores made in addition		Number of pupils	Number of crosses made in a fixed time	Number of children
5 or 6 by		1 pupil	6 or 7 by	1 girl
7 " 8 "		1 "	8 " 9 "	0 "
9 " 10 "		4 " s	10 " 11 "	4 " s
11 " 12 "		4 "	12 " 13 "	3 "
13 " 14 "		2 "	14 " 15 "	21 "
15 " 16 "		4 "	16 " 17 "	29 "
17 " 18 "		9 "	18 " 19 "	33 "
19 " 20 "		13 "	20 " 21 "	13 "
21 " 22 "		21 "	22 " 23 "	15 "
23 " 24 "		13 "	24 " 25 "	11 "
25 " 26 "		9 "	26 " 27 "	5 "
27 " 28 "		12 "	28 " 29 "	2 "
29 " 30 "		4 "	30 " 31 "	5 "
31 " 32 "		4 "	32 " 33 "	3 "
33 " 34 "		1 "	34 " 35 "	5 "
35 " 36 "		1 "	36 " 37 "	0 "
37 " 38 "		1 "	38 " 39 "	4 "
39 " 40 "		2 "	40 " 41 "	1 "
41 " 42 "		1 "		
43 " 44 "		2 "		

TABLE V.

The abilities of 6th grade girls in observing misspelled words.

Number of misspellings noticed	Number of children
10 to 14 by	1 girl
15 " 19 "	6 " s
20 " 24 "	10 "
25 " 29 "	18 "
30 " 34 "	25 "
35 " 39 "	27 "
40 " 44 "	35 "
45 " 49 "	18 "
50 " 54 "	25 "
55 " 59 "	17 "
60 " 64 "	18 "
65 " 69 "	10 "
70 " 74 "	3 "
75 " 79 "	2 "
80 " 84 "	2 "
85 " 89 "	1 "
90 " 94 "	1 "

TABLE VI.

The abilities of 4th grade girls in thinking of the opposites of words.

Score made in test with opposites	Number of children
—9 to —5 by	3 girls
—4 " 0 "	5 "
0 " 4 "	8 '
5 " 9 "	10 "
10 " 14 "	33 "
15 " 19 "	36 "
20 " 24 "	29 "
25 " 29 "	16 "
30 " 34 "	11 "
35 " 39 "	4 "
40 " 44 "	3 "

TABLE VII.

The abilities of 12 year old boys in observing letters.

Number of A's marked	Number of children
28 or 29 by	1 boy
30 " 31 "	1 "
32 " 33 "	3 " s
34 " 35 "	2 "
36 " 37 "	2 "
38 " 39 "	5 "
40 " 41 "	9 "
42 " 43 "	5 "
44 " 45 "	8 "
46 " 47 "	12 "
48 " 49 "	15 "
50 " 51 "	8 "
52 " 53 "	18 "
54 " 55 "	5 "
56 " 57 "	5 "
58 " 59 "	3 "
60 " 61 "	4 "
62 " 63 "	1 "
64 " 65 "	1 "
66 " 67 "	1 "
68 " 69 "	0 "
70 " 71 "	1 "

TABLE VIII.

The abilities of 4th grade boys in spelling.

Per cent. of words spelled correctly	Number of children
20 to 23 by	1 boy
24 " 27 "	0 "
28 " 31 "	0 "
32 " 35 "	2 " s
36 " 39 "	2 "
40 " 43 "	6 "
44 " 47 "	7 "
48 " 51 "	9 "
52 " 55 "	8 "
56 " 59 "	5 "
60 " 63 "	6 "
64 " 67 "	12 "
68 " 71 "	11 "
72 " 75 "	4 "
76 " 79 "	9 "
80 " 83 "	7 "
84 " 87 "	7 "
88 " 91 "	3 "
92 " 95 "	1 "
96 " 99 "	1 "

Individual Differences

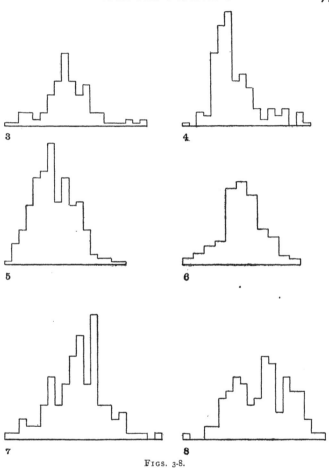

FIGS. 3-8.

FIGS. 3-8. These figures represent the facts of tables III-VIII. They are drawn after the same plan as FIG. 2 except that the sides of the columns are omitted where they are not needed to show the form of distribution.

FIG. 3 represents the abilities of 11 year olds in addition.
FIG. 4   "   "   "   " 10 year old girls in rapidity of movement.
FIG. 5   "   "   "   " 6th grade girls in observing misspelled words.
FIG. 6   "   "   "   " 4th grade girls in thinking of opposites of words.
FIG. 7   "   "   "   " 12 year boys in observing letters.
FIG. 8   "   "   "   " 4th grade boys in spelling.

76 *The Principles of Teaching*

that are most closely alike in any ability, she will yet find within that half a difference between its lowest and highest such that the latter is from one and one-fourth to one and three-fourths times as competent as the former.[1] The facts of Tables V, VI and VIII and FIGS. 5, 6 and 8 give a concrete idea of the amount of the differences be· tween children of the same grade.

The following samples of pairs of papers, each pair coming from the same class-room, tell the story of individual differences more vividly than any words or tables of figures can. These samples are in every way representative of the amount of difference to be expected in an ordinary class of even a well graded school. The classes from which they come were taken quite at random.

Two papers, A and B, written by members of the same grade and class in a test of logical power.

The questions asked were:—

1. A boy said: "I know ten good men who are doctors and ten bad men who are policemen. So doctors are better men than policemen." Did he prove it? Why? or why not?

2. If all the boys who are good in arithmetic are good in spelling, will all the boys who are good in spelling be good in arithmetic? Why? or why not?

3. A man said: "I know forty boys that studied hard and they all were promoted every year; so if you want to get rich, study hard." Was he right? Why? or why not?

4. If there was no bread or flour would everyone starve?

5. Is this true: "The more we eat, the more we grow"?

---

[1] The statements and figures of these paragraphs are by no means guesses but are made on the basis of measurements of the actual differences found by measuring the abilities of thousands of school children in a dozen or more different traits.

Individual Differences 77

6. Is this true: "If people were all blind, some women would not wear pretty dresses"?

7. If there were no schools, would children learn anything?

8. What difference would it make to people if the price of coal went up to twice what it is now?

9. Why do people send their children to school instead of making them work?

10. Which would be the worse: to have all the money in the world disappear or to have all the steel in the world disappear? Why?

A.

1. The boy did not prove it. There may be as many good policemen as there are doctors, even if he did not happen to know any.

2. No. Some boys may be able to spell well, even if they are *not* good in arith. I know from experience.

3. He was not right. The boys might have graduated from the school and yet be poor. A great many rich men have little or no education.

4. No!

5. No!

6. Yes.

7. They might.

8. People would either spend twice as much for coal as they do, or they would not use as much. They might burn wood instead, so they could probably keep warm.

9. A man or a woman with an education is a great deal better mentally and morally, and possibly physically, for they can earn their own living better when they grow up, as teachers, lawyers, doctors, etc., than they could if they chopped wood or dug in a tunnel for a living.

10. To have all the money disappear, because the whole world (or most of it) would be reduced to want and misery without money, whereas, if we have money we can make steel from iron.

B.

1. (No answer made).

2. are all good. 2. yes. because they because these question says they are

78 The Principles of Teaching

3. yes. because all that study hard will know how to make money and so get rich.

4. no

5. yes.

6. yes

7. I dont believe so

8. It would make them twice as poor as they are now and the poor of today would freez to death.

9. because they wont to fit them to work in the world when they have grown up.

10. All the money. because we need steel for building buildings and houses to live in.

Two papers, A and B, written by members of the same grade and class in a test of logical memory.

The following passage was read once and the children were asked to write the facts stated in the passage in their own or the author's words :—

Everywhere air is the first and food is the second necessity of existence.

The air we generally take for granted; but it is obviously impossible to get it pure in a town like Manchester, and very difficult to get it at all at the bottom of a mine 4,000 feet deep. This extreme depth is very rarely reached, for instance in mines near Berlin or near Prague; but it is certain that in any large town in a mining district the quality of the air both above and below ground most seriously affects the population.

Moreover, its physical effects are not the worst. In the yearly records of crime such towns occupy most unenviable positions.

A.

Air is the first and food is the second necessity for life. We generally take air for granted, but it is very difficult to obtain pure air in a town like Manchester and very hard to get at all at the bottom of a mine three or four thousand feet deep. Such depths as this are seldom reached, however, as for example the mines of Berlin and

Individual Differences 79

Moreover, lack of air is not only physically bad, but morally, for in such places the rate of crime is very high.

B.

air is not hard to get in high places but in mines and other places of the earth where the ground is low it is hard to get in the extrem it also affects the people seriously.

Two papers, A and B, written in a test like the preceding, the passage read being as follows:—

The soils of the world may roughly be divided into two great groups, according to the way the materials of that soil have been accumulated. We may have a soil which has been formed by the decaying of the rock on which it lies, or we may have a soil the particles of which have been brought from very many places and perhaps from a great distance. Of the latter group the more important are the soils carried along and finally deposited either by the rivers, the wind, or by moving ice.

A.

The soils of the world may roughly be divided into two kinds. This is partly due to the materials of which the soil is made. Sometimes it is due to the decaying of the rock on which it is. Another kind is that which has been gathered from different places by the wind, rivers or ice.

B.

The rock is sometimes deposited by moving ice sometimes by

Two translations, A and B, made by two pupils of the same grade and class (and age).

The passage to be translated was as follows:—

Atticus adolescentulus propter affinitatem P. Sulpicii, qui tribunus plebi interfectus est, non expers fuit illius periculi. Namque Anicia, Pomponii consobrina, nupserat (M.) Servio, fratri Sulpicii. Itaque interfecto Sulpicio, posteaquam vidit Cinnano tumultu civitatem esse perturbatam neque sibi dari facultatem pro dignitate

80 *The Principles of Teaching*

vivendi, quin alterutram partem offenderet, dissociatis animis civium, cum alii Sullanis, alii Cinnanis faverent partibus, idoneum tempus ratus studiis obsequendi suis, Athenas se contulit. Ac ne illa peregrinatio detrimentum aliquod afferret rei familiari, eodem magnam partem fortunarum traiecit suarum. Hic ita vixit, ut universis Atheniensibus merito esset carissimus.

Tranquillatis autem rebus Romanis remigravit Romam, ut opinor, L. Cotta et L. Torquato consulibus, quem quidem sic universa civitas Atheniensium prosecuta est, ut lacrimis desiderii futuri dolorem indicaret.

A.

Atticus a young man because of his friendship with Sulpicius, the tribune of the people who was killed was not free from this danger. For Anicia the wife of Pomponius had nursed Servius, brother of Sulpicius. And so after Sulpicius was killed and after he saw that the state was aroused by the revolt of Cinna and that no opportunity was given for him to live in accordance with his dignity without offending one or other of the parties, for the minds of the people were divided, some favoring the party of Sulla, some that of Cinna, and after he thought it was a proper time for pursuing his studies, he betook himself to Athens. And lest this migration should bring any disgrace upon his private affairs (family) he transfered a great part of his fortune to this state. Here he so lived that because of his worth he was most highly esteemed by all the Athenians (literally was most dear to all Athenians).

B.

Atticus a youth on account   of P. Sulpicus who was   a tribune of the people, was not   of his danger. And for Anicia,   of Pompey, had   , the father of Sulpicuo. And so by the killing of Sulpicius, after he saw the state to be disturbed by a tumult nor to give to himself the ability on account of his dignity, that might offend the other part, the unassociated minds of the citizens, with some Sullani other Cinnane might be favored by some   the time was followed with their desires, Athens carried itself. And lest that   some

Individual Differences 81

determination was brought to the common interest, by the same a great part of their fortune was brought. He so won that he was named the most dear to all Athens.

Two papers, A and B, written by members of the same grade and class in a test in algebra.

The test was:—
Do these examples as quickly as you can.
Do not copy them but put the work right under each example.
Take the quickest way you can to get the correct answers:

1. Simplify

$$\left(\frac{a^2-b^2}{x-y}\right)\left(\frac{x^2-y^2}{a-b}\right)\left(\frac{c^2}{x+y}\right)$$

2. What are the values of x and y if $5x + 3y = 8$ and $7x - 3y = 4$

3. A shepherd being asked how many sheep he had in his flock, said "If I had as many more, half as many more, and seven sheep and a half, I should then have 500." How many sheep had he?

4. What are the values of x and y if $1 - \frac{x+y}{x-y} = \frac{3x}{x-y}$

and $\frac{7x-3y}{23} = 3$

5. Simplify

$$\frac{\dfrac{m+n}{m-n}+\dfrac{m-n}{m+n}}{\dfrac{m-n}{m+n}-\dfrac{m+n}{m-n}}$$

6. If to the double of a certain number 14 be added, the sum is 154. What is the number?

The Principles of Teaching

A.

(1) $= c^2(a+b)$

(3) Let x = no. sheep

$x + x + \frac{1}{2}x + 7\frac{1}{2} = 500$

$2x + \frac{1}{2}x = 500 - 7\frac{1}{2}$

$2\frac{1}{2}x = 492\frac{1}{2}$

$\frac{5}{2} \times \frac{x}{\frac{747}{197}}$ $x = 197$ sheep

(2)

$12x = 12$

$x = 1$

$\therefore y = 1$

(6) Let x = Number

$2x + 14 = 154$

$2x = 154 - 14$

$x = \underline{70}$ the number

B.

(1) $\dfrac{a^2 - b^2}{x - y} \times \dfrac{a+b}{x^2 + y^2} = \dfrac{a^3 - 2ab^2 - b^3}{x^3 - 2xy^2 - y^3}$

$\dfrac{a^3 - 2ab^2 - b^3}{x^3 - 2xy^2 - y^3} \times \dfrac{c^2}{x+y} = \dfrac{a^3c^2 - 2ab^2c^2 - b^3c^2}{x^4 - 4x^2y^3 - 2xy^4 - y^9}$

(2)

$5x + 3y : 8 :: 7x - 3y : 4$

$12x : 6y :: 8 : 4$

$x : y :: 2 : 1$

$x = 2$

$y = 1$

(5) $\dfrac{\dfrac{\dfrac{m^2 - 2mn - n^2}{m^2 - 2mn - n^2}}{m^2 - 2mn - n^2}}{m^2 - 2mn - n^2} = 1.$

Individual Differences 83

Two papers, A and B, written by members of the same grade and class in a test in spelling.

A.	B.
greatful	gratful
elegant	eleagent
present	present
patience	paisionce
succeed	suckseed
severe	survere
accident	axadent
sometimes	sometimes
sensible	sensible
business	biusness
answer	anser
sweeping	swepinge
properly	prooling
improvement	improvment
fatiguing	fetging
anxious	anxchus
appreciate	apresheating
assure	ashure
imagine	amagen
praise	prasy

Principles of Teaching.—The practical consequence of the fact of individual differences is that every general law of teaching has to be applied with consideration of the particular person in question. Every stimulus must be given not to men or to children in general, but to a particular individual or group characterized by certain peculiarities. The responses of children to any stimulus will not be invariable like the responses of atoms of hydrogen or of filings of iron, but will vary with their individual capacities, interests and previous experience.

Class teaching is then always a compromise. The best stimulus for one pupil can only rarely be the best for the others. A teacher has to choose what is for the greatest good of the greatest number. He cannot expect

84 *The Principles of Teaching*

to drive forty children abreast along the highroad of education. The same responses must not be expected from all. Though obliged often to teach a class as a class, the teacher must measure the actual progress of the class by the results in each individual.

This does not at all conflict with the truth of the general laws. The law of instinct is true though children possess instincts in differing degrees of strength; the law of interest is true though children have different interests. Nor should the differences in children blind us to their likenesses. Similarity in general features is as true a fact as differences in details. Children differ greatly in their likes and dislikes, but almost all children like action and novelty. Some children like action more than others, but almost all children like it very much. Children differ greatly in their capacities, but it is safe to expect that in the great majority of cases the capacity for concrete thought will be stronger than that for abstract thought. It is folly to give up the attempt to get rational principles for teaching because the teacher's task varies with the individual to be taught. So also does the task of medicine depend on the individual to be cured, the task of agriculture on the particular crop in question. In all these three cases we need both general principles and their sagacious application to individual problems.

The worst error of teachers with respect to individual differences is to neglect them, to form one set of fixed habits for dealing with all children, to teach 'the child' instead of countless different living individuals. To realize the varieties of human nature, the nature and amount of mental differences, is to be protected against many fallacies of teaching.

A second error from which all of us suffer is to credit our scholars with natures like our own. We think

Individual Differences

of them as duplicates more or less of ourselves. If we are quick learners, we expect too much of them; if we have sensible, matter-of-fact minds, we have no patience with their sentimentalities and sensitiveness; if we are precise and neat and systematic we fail to understand how intolerable it is for them to lead a regular, orderly existence. Teachers need to add to the maxim, 'See ourselves as others see us.' the still more important one, 'See others as they are.'

§ 20. Differences in General Mental Constitution

We may profitably think of adults as men (or women) of thought, men of feeling and men of action. The scientist or inventor is typical of the first class, the poet or musician of the second, and the general or politician of the third. Of course, the complexity of human nature is so great that these classes are by no means clear and that many individuals will be prominent in two or in all three of these directions, while others will seem to belong somewhat equally well in any class. Still the division is often useful in making our judgments clear and is useful in the case of school children as well as of adults. Given any situation, some children will tend to think it out, others to respond emotionally and still others to do something. Propose to a class that instead of two sessions a day a single session lasting from nine till two be held. Some children will argue pro and con; others will cry out, 'Oh, that will be fine!' or 'I don't like that at all'; others will go to work to persuade their parents to vote in favor of one side or the other, will start petitions and the like.

Children of thought make the least difficulty in schools. Schools have been developed to suit them and teachers, being themselves commonly of that type, appre-

86 *The Principles of Teaching*

ciate their nature and needs. The teacher's mistake is more likely to be to credit all children with this general mental makeup.

Of children of feeling it may be said in the words of the nursery rhyme that when they are good they are very good indeed and when they are bad they are horrid. Nothing is more charming than the well directed enthusiasms, the bursts of noble emotion, the courage, loyalty and sympathy, the ardent responses to situations that touch the heart, of the child of this type. On the other hand, nothing is more of a nuisance than the prejudice that will not give way to fact, the sentimentality that is satisfied with feeling nobly without doing anything, the emotional excitement that passes from love to hate or from zeal to disgust on the slightest provocation. Such children are both the blessing and the bane of the teacher. Easily suggestible but hard to convince, easily aroused but easily discouraged, often brilliant but rarely steady, they require tact more than either of the other groups. The teacher's special duty to them is to direct their emotional fervor into useful channels and to teach them two great lessons: first, to judge by facts, not by their feelings, and second, to utilize every noble sentiment by acting upon it at once,—by making it a stimulus to the formation of a good habit.

To children of action the schools have been in the past least well adapted. Children often complain of school that there is nothing to do; boys who apparently get little out of school learn quickly and surely in the world of business and industry; students who could not manage their college studies, become eminent managers of men. The qualities of efficiency, cooperation and leadership in action are too important to be neglected by any teacher. Although the school is arranged specially

Individual Differences 87

for intellectual education it cannot afford to be unfair to those pupils whom nature has destined to be primarily not learners but doers. To collect samples of food from shops in the town is as good a lesson as to learn the chief products of Louisiana; to arrange for an excursion to a neighboring factory is as instructive a task as to learn the history of the invention of the cotton gin.

§ 21. *Differences in Thought*

Types of Intellect.—Individual intellects can be divided roughly into two classes: those able to work with ideas and those able to work with things. Some children manage numbers, words, parts of speech, chemical symbols and the like, but fail relatively in measuring boards, catching fish, cooking meals or making toys. They are the *idea thinkers*. Others make little headway with their arithmetic, grammar or text-book in chemistry, but succeed in the shop, the woods and the laboratory. They are the *thing thinkers*. There is, however, no opposition between these two types; indeed, a high degree of skill with ideas means a higher than average skill with things. Still for practical purposes we can classify children by their special strength into these two groups.

Schools have hitherto been managed primarily in the interest of the idea thinkers. It has been left for shops, trades and the practical activities of life to give the other group the training which their natures crave. Moreover teachers, who are likely to be of the idea thinker type are, as a consequence, likely to be unfair to the thing thinkers,—to look down on the children who do not do well in the typical school studies, however great their practical talents may be. But obviously the world needs both; the school should give opportunity for both; the

88 *The Principles of Teaching*

teacher should esteem both. To make a dynamo may not be as valuable as a preparation for college entrance examinations as to understand one; it may not be as useful a talent in the world's service. But it is one by no means to be despised. We must teach so as to help both groups.

A special class of the idea thinkers is the abstract thinkers, those who can handle not only the concrete facts of life, but also the symbols of arithmetic, algebra and geometry, the abstractly defined parts of speech and rules of syntax or the general laws of science. The abstract thinker enjoys mental gymnastics, the game of thinking regardless of the content of thought or its practical consequences. He is likely to be the pride of his teachers and to win the honors which schools give. For, just as schools and teachers commonly favor the idea thinker in comparison with the thing thinker, so they commonly favor the abstract rather than the concrete thinker. It is true that abstract power is rarer and perhaps more estimable than concrete power, but the world needs both and teachers must care for both. Practical issues, matters of mere fact, observations of nature and human life, and interests in the concrete realities of the world belong to the teacher's work as truly as do the abstract principles of language, mathematics and science.

Exceptionally Deficient Intellects.—Out of a thousand children six or eight perhaps are so stupid as to be unable to get on at all in school or to look after themselves outside of school. They are the idiots, imbeciles and the somewhat more gifted class whom we call the feeble minded. Such children should be taught in institutions or at least in special classes, but as schools are now arranged a primary school teacher is fortunate who does not in the course of a few years find in her class

Individual Differences 89

some child whose education by ordinary methods seems hopeless.

The chief defects in such children are: slowness in forming habits of any sort, lack of control of attention and, most important of all, absence of or great weakness in the capacity to think of elements or parts. This last is shown in their inability to dissociate or analyze or respond to anything other than a gross, total situation. Hence the abstract work of reading, arithmetic, science, grammar and the like is the hardest thing for them. They often can succeed with music and other technical arts and can retain concrete facts. The teacher's duty toward them when they cannot be given special education with those of their own kind, is unfailing sympathy and encouragement and a wise omission of the abstract work of the school. Enough reading and writing so that they may maintain their self-respect, enough arithmetic so that they may be able to use money intelligently, and for the rest some trade that may give them an honest living and some innocent pleasures which may give them worthy employment for their leisure—such should probably be the program for their education.

Types of Imagery.—General psychology makes us familiar with the facts that the accuracy, vividness and completeness of mental images of any sort (visual, auditory, motor, and so forth) vary greatly with individuals, and that individuals may be classed according to their capacities for getting such images at will. On the basis of these facts it is frequently recommended that teachers make their appeal in the case of any pupil through that sense whose images are strongest, that, for example, the teacher should read to the 'audiles,' have the 'motiles' copy her statement and write on the blackboard for the 'visualizers.' Plausible as this may seem, it is really

90   *The Principles of Teaching*

unwise. For in the first place, almost all pupils are of a mixed type, possessing each capacity to some degree. Hence the supposed audiles can use visual and motor images somewhat, and similarly for the supposed motiles and visualizers. In the second place the fact that a stimulus comes through one sense, say vision, does not imply that it will be remembered through an image of the same sense (here a visual image). The 'audile' or 'motile' may see words on the blackboard but have them call up non-visual images. What sense avenue is most effective for any individual does not depend on what kind of imagery he has, but upon the condition of his sense organs and his habits of attention. Children who are notable visualizers may learn better from spoken than from written words. The author of this book almost never thinks in visual images, but learns most readily from visual percepts, *i. e.*, printed words, pictures, maps, etc.

The wise course then is to arrange stimuli to appeal through several sense avenues, but to let the emphasis be on the kind of response of action or inference that the pupil makes, not upon the kind of imagery by means of which he proceeds to that response.

It is also a mistake to insist that past experiences of facts must be stored up in clear images of things, that for instance a pupil who cannot picture to his mind's eye and ear a pine forest and the roar of the surf does not know the forest and beach. It seems at first thought as if images of things rather than of words must be essential to real knowledge of things and that the clearer and more vivid the image, the more useful the knowledge; but in fact an experienced lumberman or botanist may be unable to picture a forest at all and a worker on the coast survey or a lighthouse keeper may be unable to hear in

Individual Differences 91

imagination the sound he thoroughly well knows. A man may be an eminent artist whose visualizing power is almost *nil*. One can sing a song perfectly which he cannot call up in auditory images. It is the ability to make right *responses* of thought, feeling and action that is the test of knowledge and appreciation. The essential for this is clear and vivid *experiences*, not images. It does not matter much whether the passage to the right response is through a clear or a hazy image, through images of things or images of words; not the road taken but the destination, is the important thing. It does matter somewhat, for images of things are often aids to knowledge and sources of much pleasure. The type of mind that thinks in verbal rather than thing images has however its advantages. It may feel things in memory less vividly, but it has facts about them in more convenient shape.

Although the cultivation of the capacities for imaging is hardly worth while, the methods commonly taken to cultivate them are for other reasons very useful. Thus it is an excellent exercise to have one pupil describe a tree that he has seen and let the others decide what kind of a tree it is. The value of such exercises does not, however, lie in the improvement of the capacity for imaging. In our illustration the boy who describes and the others who decide what is described may or may not base their conclusions on visual images. But they must, to describe clearly and to infer correctly from the description, know certain realities about trees. To ask a student, 'If you were a creature who could see clearly at a distance of two thousand miles and were hundreds of miles up in the air above St. Louis, what would be some of the important features that you would see to the west? To the east? To the north? To the south?';

92   *The Principles of Teaching*

to say 'Suppose that you had lived in Illinois 200 years ago, how would the country have looked, what would you have seen the inhabitants doing?'; to say, 'Think now of just how the oak leaf and the chestnut leaf look so as to tell me the difference between them,'—these are useful exercises because right responses to them mean real knowledge, but it is of little consequence what sort of images arouse the responses.

§ 22. *Differences in Action*

Types of Will.—Children, like adults, differ greatly in the extent to which some abstract quality of a situation can be made to connect with an act. Some children live almost wholly 'by special habits, not by general rules.' Tell them to use their rulers 'only in drawing figures which require accuracy' and they will ask you ten times an hour, 'Shall I use my ruler for this?' It has to be, 'Use your rulers when you draw a map. Don't use them when you draw a mountain,' etc., etc. Tell them that they may speak to one another only when it is necessary and they will whisper on the most needless occasions or, if over-scrupulous, pester you with, 'Miss ———, is it necessary for me to ask Susie Gorovitz if she wants to look at my new paint box?' and the like. Other children readily fit their acts to the abstract qualities of situations.

Children in general are much less able than adults, and very much less able than an intellectual class of adults such as teachers, to act in response to abstract elements in situations. Hence the common error in teaching is to make instructions about behavior too general and abstract, and to refer failures to follow the instructions to neglect when they are really due to incapacity.

Individual Differences

Allowance must be made in the case of those children whose wills verge toward the extreme impulsive type or toward the extreme pondering type. A teacher must not irritate the former by forever checking their natural tendency to jump at actions or the latter by hurrying them on to what seem to them impossibly hasty decisions. Too vigorous opposition to their natural bent will only make the one class confused and sulky and the other nervous and tearful. We must bring each toward the golden mean of action that is neither rash nor tardy by sympathetic and ingenious treatment. One or two concrete examples of ways and means of so doing will illustrate the right methods. Instead of saying, 'Wait! Wait! You don't know what you are about. What are you doing that for?', etc., to a pupil of the impulsive extreme, get him to agree to the simple rule that before he acts in any important situation he is to write on a bit of paper what he is going to do and why he is going to do it. At a later stage in his training have him write also why he is not going to do the opposite thing. At a still later stage have him write three or four things which might be done, the one he chooses, why he chooses to do it, and one reason for not doing each of the alternatives. Teach children of the pondering type to realize that often, when it is very, very hard to decide about an act, that very difficulty shows that it does not much matter which way one decides. Teach them that in very many cases the best course is to try one act and see how it results. 'When in great doubt, do either or both' is a maxim which these pondering children are often quite willing to follow, and which soon improves greatly the power of prompt decision. It should be their guide in all unimportant decisions and is not a bad rule for them even in really vital questions.

94   *The Principles of Teaching*

Suggestibility.—As with all other capacities there are wide differences between children in the degree of suggestibility. Ask Mary, 'Why is your work so poor to-day? Have you a headache?', and in a half hour Mary will be making more mistakes than ever and will have a headache whether she had one before or not. Ask Jane the same question in a similar situation and the reply is a prompt, 'No! Miss ———. My head is all right. I just didn't study this much.' The means of allowing for and of utilizing these differences are either too obvious to need comment or so dependent on ingenuity rather than principle as to be learnable only through practice.

§ 23. *Differences in Temperament*

The Fundamental Temperaments.—Individuals may be graded into groups with respect to the speed, vigor and range of their mental processes on scales of quick to slow, intense to weak and broad to narrow. Teaching must of course make allowance for these differences. Some first-rate thinkers are puzzled and discouraged by rapid questions or drills. Some children think and feel so intensely that they need the bit of calmness, humor and relaxation rather than the spur of excitement or rebuke. Some children cannot think of more than one thing at a time and are lost in a lesson if the teacher introduces side issues or comparative references which the broader-minded child follows easily.

The combination of slowness and weakness makes the lethargic temperament; the combination of intensity and narrowness makes the fanatic; the combination of weakness and breadth is often the basis of what we term superficiality. Of the traditional four temperaments, the *sanguine* approximates closely to the combination, quick-

Individual Differences 95

weak-broad; the *choleric* approximates closely to the combination, quick-intense-narrow; the *phlegmatic* is, of course, slow; the *melancholic* or *sentimental* is weak and commonly somewhat narrow and slow.[1]

Mental Balance.—Individuals may also be graded according to their mental balance, their ability to see things in proportion, to think and act with common sense. In little children these differences are not so obvious as they become during the high-school age. At that period it is easy to recognize the lack of mental balance shown in complaints about teachers, irregularity in school work, the presence of eccentric notions and inability to get on with parents. The lack of mental balance in parents themselves is, needless to say, one of the greatest obstacles in the teacher's path.

The Sanguine and Suspicious Types.—A practically important series of differences in temperament concerns the qualities of hopefulness and suspicion. People, even as children, differ greatly in their expectation of success and satisfaction with what is, apart from any logical basis. Some always think their affairs are to turn out well, and think whatever they do or have or see is fine; their clothes always fit them,—mentally at least,—their lessons are always well done,—in their opinion; nothing can disturb their imperturbable satisfaction. They verge toward the delusions of grandeur found in the insane. At the opposite extreme are those who always have a grudge; who feel put upon, who are ready with a tale of injustice to them; who are sure the world is a hard place. In school they are forever apologizing or sulking or complaining; in perfect kindness they see some slight; in perfect health they find some flaw. These verge toward

[1] The traditional temperaments emphasize certain emotional differences, the phlegmatic being especially hard, and the melancholic or sentimental especially easy to excite emotionally.

96 *The Principles of Teaching*

the delusions of persecution of the insane. Both groups need to learn to judge objectively by facts, not subjectively by their feelings about them. The first class must be told, 'You may feel that that is fine but nobody else thinks so; you must do your work so that it will suit the standard of others as well as your own. You are right in not being discouraged, but you are wrong in not doing your work as well as it can be done.' The second class must be told, 'No doubt you feel badly about this; but that is only because you haven't looked at it in just the right way. Nobody is against you; your judgment tells you that you have had the same chance as everyone else. Follow your judgment, not your feelings. Act as if the world was good and just and you will help make it so.'

§ 24. *Sex Differences*

In Type.—The sexes differ in mental qualities, though not so much perhaps as is generally thought to be the case. In instincts the great difference apart from the special primary instincts of sex, is in the much greater strength of the fighting instinct, of impatience of restraint and of the instinct for mastery in the male and the greater strength of the nursing, fondling instinct and of the tendencies to relieve, comfort and console in the female. In capacities no great differences between the male and female types have been demonstrated. The most marked is the female superiority in the perceptive and retentive capacities; girls, for instance, notice small details, remember lists and spell better than boys.

In Variability.—Although the male and female *types* are closely alike in intellectual capacities, there is an important difference in the deviations from the type in

Individual Differences 97

the two cases,[1] namely, that the males deviate more. The highest males in any quality are more gifted than any of the women, and the lowest males inferior to all women. Thus, though girls in general rank as high or higher than boys in high school and college, they less often lead the class; thus there are far more eminent intellects among men than among women and also twice as many idiots.

Minor Differences.—In the amount and nature of their past experiences boys and girls differ, of course, in ways too obvious to need mention. These differences are becoming less and less, however, in modern life which permits a girl to do almost everything which her brother does. Whether from native tendencies or from differences in the training of the sexes, girls are more subjective and personal, more given to judging a situation by its effect on their own feelings and affairs. They are, in the common meaning of the word, more emotional. They are somewhat neater and more accurate and somewhat less active. Their range of information and perhaps of interests is narrower. They are said to be more indirect and more deceitful. They manifest the faults of violence and insubordination less often.

SUMMARY

In any mental quality children of the same age and sex or of the same school grade, differ greatly. The distribution of amounts of any quality is such that (1) all grades from the highest to the lowest are found and that (2) mediocre amounts of it are found far more often than others, that is, that individuals center about a certain typical condition of the quality. Hence small differences are far more common than large ones.

[1] This difference is not absolutely proven to exist but it appears fairly certain from the results of several investigations.

7

98 *The Principles of Teaching*

Good teaching recognizes the variety of human nature, fits stimuli to individuals as far as possible, and, when that is not possible, chooses those stimuli which are for the greatest good of the greatest number or of the most deserving.

In particular good teaching is careful to provide for the needs of children of action, to teach children of feeling to judge by facts and to turn their good feelings into good acts, to provide for and esteem the thing thinker and the concrete thinker, to allow for different types of will and to lead each of them toward a rational balance of action.

§ 25. *Exercises*

Experiment 8. Give to forty or more pupils of the same school grade, say the sixth, two or more of the following tests :—

a. To do as many of the examples in A as possible, making as few errors as possible. Time, 2 minutes.

A.
ADDITION EXAMPLES

17	41	26	52	27	23	72	45	23	19
42	52	51	86	24	72	14	67	47	78
38	86	47	23	83	36	39	78	86	67
91	23	82	35	19	68	81	37	54	23
54	35	63	67	45	39	26	96	36	86
—	—	—	—	—	—	—	—	—	—
17	45	42	78	38	86	91	67	36	53
26	13	51	37	47	32	82	86	26	67
27	68	24	96	83	44	19	23	45	34
72	77	14	72	39	36	62	45	63	78
23	86	47	23	86	68	54	67	54	19
—	—	—	—	—	—	—	—	—	—

Individual Differences

b. To spell the following words from dictation:—

wrong	therefore	grateful	appreciate
young	praise	anxious	thoroughly
rough	properly	imagine	conscientious
cheap	present	realize	millinery
asleep	exception	experience	necessary
running	patience	occasion	
slipped	elegant	delicious	
straight	sweeping	triumph	
noisy	peculiar	intelligent	
thought	importance	character	
sometimes	succeed	approval	
pleasure	severe	ascending	
difference	accident	possess	
answer	sensible	physician	
business	assure	Massachusetts	

c. To write beside each word in list C. 1 a word meaning the opposite, 'meaning just what the word you see does not mean.' Time, 60 seconds; skipping to be allowed. Repeat the test using C. 2.

C. 1		C. 2	
like	good	north	great
rich	outside	open	hot
sick	quick	round	dirty
glad	tall	sharp	heavy
thin	big	east	late
empty	loud	known	first
war	white	something	left
many	light	stay	morning
above	happy	push	much
friend	false	nowhere	near

d. Read each of these sentences. If what it says is true, put an *r* after it. If what it says is false, put a *w* after it. Time, 15 minutes.

1. If all children could learn their lessons without help there would be no use in having schools.

2. Boys may eat a great deal and grow only a little, they may eat very little and grow a great deal.

The Principles of Teaching

3. Growing richer sometimes means growing unhappier.

4. In the summer vacation we have a good time but we don't learn anything.

5. New York has become the largest city in the United States because it was settled so early.

6. The reason why agriculture is more important than manufactures is that it is healthier to work on a farm than in a factory.

7. It would be better to have all the gold and silver in the world disappear than to have all the iron disappear.

8. The rates for passengers and freight from Cincinnati to New Orleans by boat ought to be cheaper than by train.

9. If you add nine thirteens together you get 117.

10. A man has $963 and needs 1500 dollars. He must get $567.

11. If I mix 8 quarts of water with 12 quarts of milk, forty fourths of the mixture will be milk.

12. If I have to carpet a room which is 10 by 13 feet and have already a border a foot wide around it I must buy 12 square yards of carpet.

Mark each addition paper by giving 1 for each half example done and 2 for each half example that is correct, or by any other reasonable method.

Mark each spelling paper by giving 1 for each word spelled correctly.

Mark each 'opposites' paper by giving 1 for each correct opposite, .5 for doubtful ones.

Mark each 'logic' paper by giving 1 for each correct answer and taking off 1 for each sentence marked incorrectly.

When the papers are scored, make out for each test a table showing how many children scored 0; how many, 1; how many, 2; how many, 3; how many, 4; and so on. Make also for each test a statement telling the average ability found, the ability found most frequently, the total range of ability found, the limits between which the

Individual Differences 101

abilities of about half of the children lie, the limits between which about three-fourths lie.

Experiment 9. Ask thirty or more individuals, boys and girls in their teens preferably, but adults if more convenient, to mark with a (1) the occupation which they like best of the ten below, with a (2) the one they like next best, and so on. Cases where the individual has not had enough experience of the thing in question to enable him to tell how well he would like it may be marked (?). How much agreement is there?

Being present at a party.
Eating a good dinner.
Playing indoor games, such as games of cards.
Playing outdoor games, such as baseball, basket ball, tennis.
Working with tools, as in carpentering or gardening.
Hearing music, as at a concert.
Being present at the theatre.
Reading a story.
Resting, such as lying in a hammock or on a couch.
Travelling or seeing new places.

Write a brief account of the results of Experiments 8 and 9, telling especially how they illustrate the statements of this chapter.

1. Which would commonly be better, for all of a class to engage in a review, or for some to be given outside reading instead?

2. Should all pupils engage in every recitation, or should some be given special 'seat-work'?

3. What would you suggest as language work for pupils whose habits are already perfect with respect to the usage that is being taught to the class in general?

4. What would you suggest as work during a reading lesson in Latin or German for those pupils who are sure to know how to translate the lesson very well? What would be the advantage in having them write out a

102 *The Principles of Teaching*

free translation in as good English as they could? In having them read and write a summary of some book or article about Roman life or German life? In giving them the time to use as they liked?

5. (a) What could probably be wisely omitted from the arithmetic work of say a seventh grade in the case of the pupils least gifted in arithmetic? (b) Answer the same question in the case of grammar for those least gifted in grammar. (c) In the case of algebra (in the first year of high school) for those least gifted in algebra.

6. (a) Theoretically, should all pupils take the same studies? (b) Should all pupils do the same work in any one study? (c) When all are given the same work, should all be expected to reach the same degree of skill?

7. Criticise the practice revealed in this school announcement: 'The diploma of the school is awarded to all those who have completed satisfactorily the entire course. Pupils will be excused from no part of it on account of sickness, accident, lack of earnestness or inability.' [23]

8. 'It is generally conceded by educators that all classification in schools should be based upon reading and arithmetic, the former in the lower grades, and the latter in all the more advanced classes.' [24] What is the objection to the common practice described in this quotation? State a method of classification for the grammar grades that would be theoretically better than that on the basis of arithmetic and equally practicable.

9. Mention three or four ways in which you would vary your methods of teaching to make them fit a girl who was a child of feeling, with superior capacity to work with ideas, impulsive and suggestible.

10. How would you vary them to fit a boy who was

Individual Differences 103

a child of action, with superior capacity to work with things?

11. How would you vary them to fit a boy who was a thinker, especially with ideas, quick and sanguine, with poor mental balance?

12. Make a list of ten men and women whom you and some of your friends know well, say of ten fellow students.

(a) Characterize each of them as a man (or woman) of action, of feeling or of conduct, and as thing thinker or idea thinker.

(b) Rank the ten in each of the following traits:
> Capacity to act in response to partial aspects of facts.
> Impulsiveness of will.
> Suggestibility.
> Quickness.
> Intensity.
> Breadth.
> Hopefulness.

Score the highest one of the ten 1, the next highest 2, the next highest 3, the middle four M, the lowest 10, the next lowest 9, and the second from the lowest 8. A table like that given below will be convenient.

RANK IN

Individual	Partial Activity	Impulsive- ness	Suggest- ibility	Quick- ness	Intensity	Breadth	Hopeful ness
A							
B							
C							
D							
E							
F							
G							
H							
I							
J							

Unfortunately there can be no sure and easy veri-

104 *The Principles of Teaching*

fication of the correctness of such judgments of character as these. It is interesting however to compare one's own judgments with the averages of the marks given by the four or five best judges of character in the class.

13. How would you explain the fact that though girls have on the average as good intellects as boys, the latter do better at such intellectual games as chess and whist?

14. It is commonly said, and is probably true, that girls do not cooperate as well as boys. Bearing in mind the qualities upon which cooperation depends, which sex difference of those mentioned might account for the fact?

15. How can it be that there are so many more great writers, inventors and scientists among men than among women if in average capacity the sexes are alike?

16. Would you expect the most interesting pupils to be more frequently of the male or of the female sex? Why?

Experiment 10. With the help of friends or classmates get from fifty or more teachers' answers to these questions: 'What is the name of the most interesting pupil you ever had? What is the name of the brightest? What is the name of the worst (morally)?' What is the result? Does it justify your expectation expressed in the answer to question 16?

17. Are boys or girls the more likely to interpret a teacher's criticisms as the result of a grudge against them?

For Further Reading

E. A. Kirkpatrick, *Fundamentals of Child Study,* Chapter XVI.

J. Adams, *Herbartian Psychology Applied to Education,* Chapter 1V.

J. MacCunn, *The Making of Character,* Chapter III.

CHAPTER VII

ATTENTION

Preparatory, *Elements of Psychology,* §§ 19 and 59

§ 26. *Instinct and Habit and Attention*

When and how a pupil attends is a matter of instinct and habit; there is no royal road to winning attention, but only the regular highway through the development of interest and the reward of acts of attention by some increment of satisfaction to the pupil. The principles of teaching with reference to attention are all implied in the chapter on interests and in a chapter to come on habit. There is no need to repeat them. Some corollaries of these principles may, however, be briefly mentioned.

Inattention commonly means attention to something else; only rarely does a teacher have to struggle with general· mental apathy, utter absence of focalized thinking. The common battle is between the stimulus he gives and some competitor; the teacher's task is to outbid some rival. Attention is not a quantity to be created, but a force to be directed.

Attention is not secured by demanding it. The demand for attention avails only if, in the pupil's experience, obeying the demand has brought satisfaction or if disobeying it has brought discomfort. To demand attention without soon arousing real interest will result in the connection, 'attention given when asked—a dull, unpleasant half-hour.'

106   *The Principles of Teaching*

To gain attention is not to hold it. The former is comparatively easy and also comparatively unimportant. Although the habit of immediate response to whatever signals are used to attract attention should be firmly fixed, it is after all only a minor means to efficient work. In fact, if a school day includes a long succession of devices to win back the attention of the pupils, it means a superficial ingenuity rather than fundamentally right methods of teaching. Steady attention through interests and the habit of work is the desideratum.

It is not enough to simply have attention; it must be attention to the right thing. As was said in Chapter V, a lecturer on the sequence of tenses can easily get the attention of his audience by telling a funny story, but the chances are ten to one that the attention will not be to the sequence of tenses. Showing pictures, relating anecdotes, playing games and the like may even, if used carelessly, distract attention from its proper object. To get attention but to something other than the fact to be learned or act to be done is as bad as to have a pupil remember but remember the wrong answer.

One means to secure attention is to secure its physical attitude. If sitting up straight and looking at the teacher has gone with attention oftener than has lolling back and wriggling, then the attention of a lolling class can be improved by having them sit up straight. If we need to study a book, we can at least open it and look at the words. Interest may come then which would fail to come so long as we sat thinking, 'I ought to study that lesson.' Teachers need to remember, however, that attention as measured by results and not some special bodily attitude is the essential. Efficient attention is possible with all sorts of bodily attitudes, and on the other hand

Attention   107

children readily learn to mimic the postures of attention, without having the reality.

§ 27. *Exercises*

Clearness, intensity, novelty (but with sufficient familiarity to be grasped), pleasurableness and expectedness are qualities which in and of themselves attract attention to the stimulus possessing them.

1. Of these six qualities, which is always desirable as a feature of the stimuli given by a teacher?

2. Which two lose their effect with use?

3. Which offers an argument for stating the aim of each lesson?

4. Which explains why a rough drawing is often preferable to an expensive picture or map?

5. What is the objection to the following method of securing attention?

'The pupil reads until the teacher says, "next," when the next in turn commences at the exact word (or part of a word) where the former ceased, or forfeits his place in the class.' [25]

6. What is the objection to repeating a question?

7. Compare the two spelling lessons below with respect to their efficiency in securing attention to the essentials.

A.	blue	blew	
	sea	see	
	their	there	
	knew	new	
B.	blue	blew	The sky is blue. The wind blew.
	to	two	too
	sea	see	Ships sail on the sea. You see with your eyes.

108 *The Principles of Teaching*

their	there	He gave them their books. He went there to-day.
knew	new	The girl knew the lesson. Put on your new hat.
to two too		He went to school with his two brothers. His sister went too.

8. What would be the advantage of giving also as models or as sentences to be written?

> Red, blue and green are common colors.
>
> He has his book, her book and your book.
>
> Fred and Mary have their books.
>
> Where is he? Is he here? No! He is there.

9. Recitations are often so conducted that if a scholar already knows his lesson he gains nothing from the recitation. What is the result?

10. If a scholar regards reciting as primarily a means of testing the knowledge of the one reciting, how often will he attend during the recitation?

11. What would you do to make attention to the answers of other pupils bring 'some increment of satisfaction to each pupil'?

12. How would arranging with parents for the provision of a separate room for study (or at least a corner with table and lamp) improve the home work of pupils?

13. What would be the effect upon pupils' attention of peculiarities of appearance, dress and manners in the teacher?

Experiment 11. Turn over twenty or twenty-five pages of the advertising section of a magazine rapidly. Record the things which caught your attention by recording those which you remember. Use an English magazine so as not to measure knowledge rather than attention. Have two or more children do likewise (the more, the better). How do your records illustrate the facts stated

Attention 109

in the first paragraph of this section? How do they illustrate the nature of children's interests?

For Further Reading

W. James, *Talks to Teachers on Psychology*, Chapter XI.

J. Adams, *Herbartian Psychology Applied to Education*, Chapter VI.

CHAPTER VIII

Principles of Association

Preparatory, *Elements of Psychology,* §§ 43-50

§ 28. *Habit Formation*

The general law of association answered the question, 'How may the teacher choose stimuli that will produce the desired present response?', by the principle of apperception. The same law answers the question, 'How may the teacher arrange stimuli, so as to insure right responses in the future?', by the principles of habit formation.

It is a fundamental law of mental life that if a mental state or bodily act is made to follow or accompany a certain situation with resulting satisfaction it will tend to go with that situation in the future. The applications of the law to teaching are comprised in the simple and obvious, but too commonly neglected rules. *Put together what you wish to have go together. Reward good impulses.* Conversely; *Keep apart what you wish to have separate. Let undesirable impulses bring discomfort.*

Obvious as these rules are to the student of human nature, they are constantly violated. For instance, the commonest school punishment of the writer's school-days was to keep pupils in school over-time, thus putting the idea of punishment, of undesirability, into closest connection with the experience of school and school work.

Principles of Association

The old methods of teaching reading connected the sight of the letters with the sounds of their names, b a d being thus put with bee ay dee and d o g with dee oh gee. The writer was taught in Latin to connect *amabat* only with *amabam, amabas* in front of it and *amabamas, amabatis* after it. What wonder that it did not call up in his mind 'he was loving'!

Still more flagrant are the violations of the law, *Reward good impulses.* The mother neglects her children when they are quiet and decent and plays with them only when they cry. Consequently there are many crying babies. The child is refused a favor when he asks once, but if he teases a score of times it is finally granted. Consequently there are many teasing boys.

The mind does not gravitate toward truth, wisdom and goodness of its own accord. What it does is to keep together those ideas, feelings and acts which it experiences together and with resulting satisfaction. If a situation is to call up its proper response, that response should be put with that situation in the individual's experience. The mind does not do something for nothing. If it is to drop one tendency and cherish another, the latter must be made the more satisfying. To get habits we must make them and reward them. *Put together what you wish to have go together. Reward good impulses.*

As in the case of apperception, the principle of habit formation is fully treated in dynamic psychology. All that is required here is training in its special applications through appropriate exercises. I venture, however, to remind the reader that the general law of association applies to every form of connection, to connections of impression and expression as well as to connections between one idea and another. Hence the laws of teach-

112 *The Principles of Teaching*

ing derived from it apply to sense-training, observation, attention, bodily skill, behavior, morality, emotional responses, aesthetic appreciation, interests and ideals as well as to memory and thought.

§ 29. Exercises

1. Why do little children give such definitions as the following?

A lunch is when you go to the woods.

Coffee is what old folks drink.

2. Why do they define an object by its use far oftener than by its structure?

3. Do you believe the following? A boy in reciting said, 'The sailor was sorry that he done it.' The teacher said, 'What are the principal parts of *to do?*' The boy said, 'Do, did, done.'

4. In what connection does a pupil need to feel 'came' rather than 'comed,' 'brought' rather than 'bringed' or 'brang,' and the like? How would you teach the principal parts of verbs?

5. Name one advantage which written work has over oral as a method of learning spelling.

6. Which of these four procedures is the best? Why?

(a) A teacher prints a, b, c, d, e, etc., on the board and, pointing at each in turn, gives the name,—ay, bee, see, dee, eee, eff, etc.

(b) A teacher prints red on the board, and, pointing at each letter in turn, says, 'arr, ee, dee, red.'

(c) A teacher prints 'red' on the board and, pointing at it, says, 'red.'

(d) A teacher calls attention to a maple leaf that has turned and says, 'What color is this leaf?' The answer

Principles of Association

being given, she says, 'I will say its color with the chalk,' and saying, 'This leaf is,'—prints or writes, 'red.'

7. Should the beginner in Latin learn adjectives as in (a) or as in (b) or as in (c)?

(a)			(b)	(c)
bonus	a	um	bonus	vir bonus
boni	ae	i	boni	viri boni
etc.			bono	. .
			etc.	. .
				. .
				. .
				puella bona
				puellae bonae,
				etc.

8. What connections of impression are made in the following exercises in correcting misspellings?

"1. Nolledje is the best foundashun ov happenes. It distingwishes sivilized from savidje life. Its kultevashun in yuth promotes vertshu, bi kreating habits ov menttal disseplin; and bi inkulkating a sense ov morral oblegashun.

2. Man is an anemal endoued with pouers ov kommunikashun, memmury, assosheashun, immetashun, refleckshun, and rezoning; talents given him bi hiz Makur; for the good use ov witsh, he is akkountabel in a futshure state.

3. Man, in his unimprooved and unsivilized kondishun is naked, without habetashun, without menes ov defense or offense, and pozzessed ov no menes ov subsistense, besidez the wild froots and spontaneus prodduse ov the erth.

4. Menny nashuns, evn now, liv nakid in kavurns undur ground, purform no labur, and depend for thare subsistense on the spontaneus produkts ov the erth, and on the flesh ov anemals, witsh tha destroy bi simple strattajems.

5. The oridjenal inhabittants ov the Amerikan kon-

The Principles of Teaching

tenent lived nakid, paneted thare boddys ov vareus kullurs, bestoed littel or no kultevashun on the soil, and depended for subsistense on akorns, berres, and roots, and uppon thare skil and sukses in hunting and fishing." [26]

"'Tis the last rose of sumer left bloomin alone,
  All its lovly compannions are faded and gone;
  No flour of its kindrid, no rosebud is nye,
  To refflect back its blushes and return sie for sie.
  I'll not leeve thee, thou loan one, to pyne on the stemm,
  Sinse the lovly are sleaping, go sleap thou with them.
  Thus kindly I skatter thy leafs o'er the bead,
  Where thy mates of the garden lye senceless and ded."
                                                   [27]

9. How would you modify the statement, 'Practice makes perfect'?

10. (a) Name two or three school punishments which put the feeling of undesirability with things with which teachers should not wish it to go. (b) In what cases may neglect of a pupil's bad behavior be a better deterrent than a rebuke?

11. Give three or four illustrations from home or school life of training that rewards actually bad impulses.

12. What habit is formed by echo questions, such as, 'Washington was at Valley Forge. Where was Washington?' 'The citizens rose in their might and conquered the invader. What did the citizens do?'

13. Justify the following recommendations on the basis of the law of habit-formation:—

Make no rules that you cannot enforce.

Make no laws infringements of which you cannot detect.

14. Suppose that after the events related in the following some one had asked the girl if she would like to go to heaven where she could look at God, how would she have felt?

Principles of Association 115

WANTING TO SEE GOD.

"One day Clara and Willy went with their mother to walk in the fields. They were much pleased to see the pretty flowers and to hear the birds sing. 'Oh,' said Willy, 'how great God is! He must be very lovely. How I would like to see him!' 'And so would I,' said Clara, 'if it were only for half a minute.' 'I am afraid,' said their mother, 'You could not look at Him. He is so bright, you could not bear the sight.' 'Oh,' said Willy, 'we like to look at things that are bright. Mama, please do let us see God.' 'Well,' said their mother, 'now look at the sun for half a minute and tell me what you see.' Their eyes followed their mother's finger as she pointed to the sun, which was just breaking through the clouds. 'Oh, oh,' they both cried, 'it hurts our eyes; it dazzles us so, we cannot look at it.' 'Well', said their mother, 'the glory of God is so great, that in His presence the sun would seem dark. But if you are good and love Him, you will one day see Him and be happy with Him in heaven.'" [28]

15. What should be connected with the sight of a letter of the alphabet?

16. Which is the more necessary connection with the sight of a word, its sound or its meaning?

17. Which general feeling do we wish to have connected with reading lessons in the scholar's mind, that printed and written words are 'things to be said when you see them' or 'things that tell you something'?

18. Name two or more advantages of the following method for the first few weeks in reading:—[1]

Large cards are arranged with *The door, A window, The table, A book, Fred, Dan* and other names of the children in the class, *walks, runs, stands still* and the like printed or written on them in large letters.

The teacher says, 'This is Fred, so we will put a card

[1] Recall the principles of instinct and interest as well as those of habit formation.

116   *The Principles of Teaching*

on him that says *Fred* so that we will all know.   I am the teacher and this card says *Teacher*,' fastening it to her dress.   'Would you like a card that tells your name, Dan?   All right, here is Dan's name,' fastening it to Dan.   (And so on through all or part of the class.) 'Mary and Alice and Fred may stand here with me.' Pointing to Mary's label, 'What does this say?'   Similarly with *Alice, Fred* and *teacher*.   Then, taking off the four cards and standing them up before the class.   'Mary, can you find your card?   Alice, find yours.   Fred, please bring me mine.   Whose card is this?' (taking the one left).   Putting the cards back in a row before the class, 'Henry may put Dan's card on Dan.   Who can put Mary's card on Mary?   Nellie may.   We will let Fred get his own.   Get yours, Fred.   What does this one say?' (taking the one left).

'Shall we give the table a card?   Isaac may hang the table's card on the front of the table.   It says, *The table.* This says, *The door.*   Where shall we put it?   Yes, you may, Lawrence.   What else in the room shall have a card with its name on it?   Yes, the picture-book can have one.   This says, *a book.*   Stand it up by the book, Mary Dorgan.   Who can find the card that says, *the table?*   Bring it to me.'   Ditto with *the door, a book.* Standing the cards for *teacher, Fred, Mary, Alice, the table, the door,* and *a book* in a row, the children are allowed to find the one that says *teacher,* etc.

19.   If you accept the principle that in the first month of reading, direct connections should be made between the sight of the words and realities, how would you teach such words as *runs, run, stands still, stand still?*

20.   How would you teach *on, in, around?*

21.   In using printed cards in the way just described, what would be the gain of leaving each card fastened to

Principles of Association 117

its object in the interval between one reading lesson and another?

22. If every person in a family always wore his name, if the furniture, the utensils and toys of the house were all clearly labelled and a child was rewarded for every chance attention to and recognition of the labels, what would happen?

23. What is the reward for reading in ordinary life?

24. What objection is there to telling the story to a class before they read it?

25. What advantage might there be in having the children ask in writing for the little favors which they wish?

26. When a child learns to say off *one, two, three, four, five, six, seven, eight, nine, ten,* just what connections are formed?

27. What connections are formed when he learns to count by pointing at each one of a group of objects in order and saying one, two, three, four, and so on as he points?

28. What undesired connection may be formed when the teacher, after displaying four leaves and asking, 'How many?', takes another leaf, puts it with the four, saying, 'How many now?', and elicits the answer, 'Five'?

29. Which of the charts reproduced in Figs. 9 and 10 would you prefer to use in teaching beginning arithmetic? Why?

30. The application of arithmetical principles ought of course to be connected with problems of actual experience both in order to waste no effort and in order to strengthen the connection 'arithmetic—of real use in the world.' Replace each of the following by a better problem which gives the same drill but does not violate the principle just stated.

a. 'Bought $\frac{6}{7}$ of a box of candles, and having used $\frac{7}{8}$ of them, sold the remainder for $\frac{16}{25}$ of a dollar: how much would a box cost at the same rate?   Ans. 5\frac{13}{15}$.' [29]

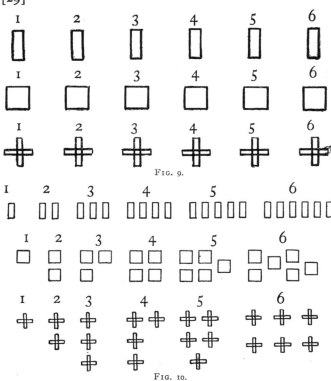

FIG. 9.

FIG. 10.

b. 'Allowing that 4 persons can stand on one square rod, how many persons can stand on one acre?' [30]

c. 'Divide a quantity of tea weighing 51 lbs. 1 oz. amongst a man, a woman and a boy, giving the man twice the woman's share, and the woman thrice the boy's share.' [31]

Principles of Association 119

d. 'A man had nine dozen eggs in a basket. He sold one shilling's worth at a half-penny each; then sixpenny worth at four for three pence. He put 27 fresh eggs into his basket and sold four score; a dozen and a half got broken. How many eggs had he left at last?' [32]

31. An eminent student of teaching, Mr. Adams of London, is quoted as objecting strongly to the practice, common amongst men teachers in England, of wearing black clothes in the school-room. How might he support his criticism?

32. In what places does this lesson put together things which do not logically go together?

Dog.

What is this?

The dog.

For what is the dog useful?

He is a faithful servant to man; and, as he is permitted to accompany him, he feels proud; and, above all other animals, he is useful to defend his master's person and property.

Does the dog know more than most other animals?

He does; he loves and obeys his master, and always does as he is bid. [33]

33. (a) If a marksman never saw where his shots hit, how rapidly would his aim improve? (b) If examinations are given, should the pupil be told his degree of success? (c) How can this be done without encouraging too much attention to a pupil's success compared with that of others in the same class? (d) Should his papers be returned to him? (e) Should only his errors be commented on?

34. Apply the facts of the law of association to teaching irregular plurals.

35. To teaching the conjugations in Latin.

120   *The Principles of Teaching*

36. To teaching dates in history.

37. Should the tables in arithmetic be built up gradually from knowledge gained elsewhere of the individual associations which they contain or be given once and for all as a total orderly system? Why?

38. Into what units would you divide a dictation in reading it to a class? Would you, for instance, give one word at a time or four words at a time? Mark the places where you would make pauses in dictating (A) to a third-year class and in dictating (B) to a seventh-year class.

(A) A shepherd saw that a wolf had, for many days, been near his sheep. The wolf had in no way tried to kill any of them. But the shepherd did not like to see a wolf near by.

(B) To the Boys of America.

"Of course what we have a right to expect from the American boy is that he shall turn out to be a good American man. Now, the chances are strong that he won't be much of a man unless he is a good deal of a boy. He must not be a coward or a weakling, a bully, a shirk or a prig. He must work hard and play hard. He must be clean-minded and clean-lived, and able to hold his own under all circumstances and against all comers. It is only on these conditions that he will grow into the kind of a man of whom America can really be proud. In life as in a football game the principle to follow is: Hit the line hard; don't foul and don't shirk, but hit the line hard." [34]

39. Does or does not the connection between the thought of a situation and the thought of an act imply that when the thought appears the act will be made?

40. Does or does not the connection between an idea

Principles of Association

121

of an event and an idea of a certain emotion imply that when the event takes place, the emotion will be felt?

41. If you wish to be *sure* that whenever the alarm-clock rings you will always get out of bed, what must you do?

42. What do your answers to questions 39, 40 and 41 suggest about moral training?

43. James gives as rules for making habits the following: "We must take care to launch ourselves with as strong and decided an initiative as possible. Never suffer an exception to occur till the new habit is securely rooted in your life. Seize the very first possible opportunity to act on every resolution you make, and on every emotional prompting you may experience in the direction of the habits you aspire to gain." [35]

Illustrate these rules in the case of forming the habit of punctuality.

44. Give two cases where the right and thé wrong habits are equally or nearly equally easy to form.

45. Which is much more important in such cases, the starting of the habit or the same amount of training later?

46. What do your answers to Questions 44 and 45 suggest (a) concerning the first steps in learning the pronunciation of a foreign language? (b) Concerning the quality of the voice of teachers in primary schools?

47. What danger is to a considerable extent avoided by arranging a series of easy propositions for the beginning of a course in geometry and requiring them to be done as originals?

48. The capacity to break away from one habitual series of connections, to do things in an unfamiliar way, is important; mere machine-like performance of certain acts is deadening. Hence some teachers infer that to

122   *The Principles of Teaching*

make any connection perfect through practice arrests the development of originality. Give evidence that it is, on the contrary, a better preventive of deadening routine to make connections sure but to make many of them, than to give little drill on any.

49. What additions should then be made to the following statements to make them valid? The passing of papers, pens, books and the like should be done as the result of mechanical habit, but—

50. Knowledge of the arithmetical tables should be made into perfect habits, but these habits must be—

Experiment 12. Give to a third grade test A, starting all the pupils at the same time and stopping them the moment any one finishes. A day or so later give test B, allowing the same time as for A. Compare the number of examples done correctly in the two cases. Explain the differences.

A.

1. Divide by 6 the number 36.
2. What number divided by 3 will give 11?
3. What number must be added to 42 to make 85?
4. From what number must 28 be taken to leave 59?

B.

1. Divide 28 by 4.
2. How much is 12 times 4?
3. Subtract 24 from 58.
4. Add 82 and 95.

Experiment 13. Teach one or more first grade or kindergarten children the combinations, *three and two are five, three and four are seven, three and five are eight, three and six are nine,* without giving them any statements about *two and three, four and three, five and three* or *six and three.* After the three and two, three and four, etc., are well mastered, test each child with the

Principles of Association 123

combinations, asking now for three and five, now for six and three and so on with a mixture of both orders. To which order are the responses more often correct?

§ 30. *Memory*

Associative memory, memories of facts *in their connections,* is what memory means in discussions of teaching. Such memories are simply habits due to the general law of association or connection-forming; the principles of teaching so as to secure such memories quickly, surely and permanently are results of the general law as applied to those connections between word and meaning, thing and name, numbers and their sum, event and date, one line of a poem and the next, name of law and detailed statement of law and the like, which we think of under the term, memory. If one thing is to call another to mind, the second must be connected with the first often or energetically and the pupil must be rewarded for connecting them. If facts are to call others to mind when they are needed, the connections must be arranged in useful systems.

As a rule it is more economical to put things together energetically than to put them together often; close attention is better than repetition. The active recall of a fact from within is, as a rule, better than its impression from without; for recall is a helpful way to be sure of close attention and also forms the connection in the way in which it will later be required to act. Furthermore, if children are taught to memorize by recall, they are saved from wasting time in reading over and over or studying at length facts which they have already committed to memory. In memorizing by recall one not only knows a fact; he also knows when he knows it.

124   *The Principles of Teaching*

It is fashionable nowadays to decry memory as a sort of cheap slavey of the intellect, a 'skeleton in the closet' of teaching, not fit to be mentioned in the polite society of apperception, interest, reasoning and the rest. In the laudable effort to cure school work of the error of trusting everything to verbal memory, writers on teaching have made the mistake of the surgeon who cured a sprained ankle by cutting off the leg.

Indeed the trouble was not with memory, but with what was remembered,—words only. We surely must not cut a man's legs off, because he walks into danger on them! If a fact is understood, the better it is remembered, the better off we are. It does little good to explain a process so skillfully as to make it perfectly understood, if the explanation has to be repeated again the next week or day. Moreover there is and probably always will be in school work a great bulk of fact which pupils can understand without any difficulty, but which can be made their permanent possession only by definite effort.

§ 31. *Exercises*

There are three common ways of memorizing, by repetition, concentration, and recall.

1. Which is the one commonly used by children?

2. Which is the one commonly advocated by teachers?

3. Which is the best? Why?

4. Ebbinghaus found that it took sixteen repetitions to learn a series of twelve nonsense syllables, and fifty-five repetitions to learn a series of twenty-six. What suggestion would you get from this concerning memorizing poems, model sentences, quotations, etc.?

5. Miss Aiken found that a poem could be best

Principles of Association 125

learned by first learning a skeleton of the leading words, verbs, etc. What suggestion would you get from this concerning learning about a period in history or a topic in geography?

6. Just what was the fault of the method of teaching represented by the following announcement of the work of the junior class in a New England school in 1826?

"From nine, to about ten o'clock.

Junior Class.—The pupils are occupied in writing on their slates prepared copies, or paragraphs from the orthographical exercises, or the lesson previously committed to memory in Grammar or Geography.

From ten, to about eleven o'clock.

The pupils are occupied in pronouncing and spelling three columns of words with the book, very distinctly, four times. After which, they read in Murray's Reader (the first and second parts alternately).

From eleven, to twelve o'clock.

The pupils are occupied in writing a copy. After which, they commit to memory a lesson in Grammar or Geography, and the spelling already enunciated. Before they are dismissed, they are required to recite the same distinctly and accurately.

From two, to about three o'clock.

The pupils are occupied in spelling as in the morning. After which, they read in the Bible or New Testament.

From three, to about four o'clock.

The pupils are occupied in ciphering.

From four, to five o'clock.

The pupils are occupied in writing a copy. After which (if a sufficient portion of ciphering is completed), they commit to memory the spelling already enunciated, and before they are dismissed, they are required to recite the same distinctly and accurately." [36]

7. "No invention of man has as yet been able to supersede the pen as the primary exponent of thought, and its use, instead of being confined to the few, as in

126 *The Principles of Teaching*

time past, is now essayed to be taught to every individual.

Upon it rests the whole superstructure of commerce and literature, while it furnishes the readiest and most reliable means for correspondence of every kind.

Has any invention of man been able as yet to dispense with the pen? What is said of its universal use? What rests upon the use of the pen?" [37]

What is the relation between the type of questions given above and the following type of answer: 'Commerce and manufactures is the governor of the state and George Wolf the occupation of the people of Pennsylvania.'

8. Which of the following questions encourage mere verbal memory?

9. Which of them encourge guessing at the expense of inference or frank confession of ignorance?

10. Which of them form associations meaningless outside of the lesson-hour at the expense of really valuable connections?

11. Which of them form associations which are actually harmful?

    a. What of the Atlantic?

    b. What of Queen Isabella?

    c. What had Christopher Columbus done?

    d. Might a war have resulted from this?

    e. What preparations were made? (The text with which this question goes reads, 'They even made preparations to resist by force of arms.')

    f. What do they take up in church after the prayer (asked in the course of an effort to explain, 'Any collection of units is expressed by a whole number')?

    g. What will soon be seen?

    h. Was this successful? (The assault on Petersburg of June, 1864.)

Principles of Association   127

    i. Has his example been followed?

    j. Who dragged whom around the walls of what city?

    k. The text reading, 'Glass is transparent,' the question is asked, 'Why can you see through glass?'

    l. What did the English still do?

    m. The text reading, 'Everybody in the colony had been talking of the independence of the colonies,' the question is put, 'What had the people been talking of?'

    n. What proposal was made and by whom?

    o. Was the offer accepted?

12. In the light of the classification just made, (a) state an objection to using the words of a text-book in framing a question about its subject-matter. (b) State also a risk incurred in asking any question which has meaning only in a particular context.

§ 32. *Correlation*

Just as the business of teaching is not only to impart ideas but also to connect them with one another in useful habits of thought, so also its business is not to stop at a multitude of single habits unconnected with each other, but to connect these again into useful systems with useful cross-connections between systems. Just as one idea should be related to another with which it ought to go, so one series of connected ideas should be related to others with which it ought to go.

The group of mental connections which we call knowledge of percentage should connect with the group which we call knowledge of decimal fractions on the one hand and with the group which we call knowledge of

128 *The Principles of Teaching*

interest on the other. Knowledge of the climate of Central America should connect with knowledge of the general facts about Central America's latitude, elevation, prevailing winds and the like, with knowledge of the general laws of climate and with knowledge of the manner of life of the inhabitants of Central America. The problems of high-school physics should connect with knowledge of algebra as well as with knowledge of certain physical laws.

The principle that knowledge should be not a multitude of isolated connections, but well-ordered groups of connections, related to each other in useful ways,—should not be a hodge-podge of information, but a well-ordered system whose inner relationships correspond to those of the real world,—is called the principle of *Correlation*. It implies that lesson and lesson be brought into relations one with another in a larger unit of some one general topic, that one topic be brought into relations with another in a still larger unit, and that one subject of study be taught with reference to the other subjects whenever the facts they present have important bearings one upon the other in the real world.

The method of securing such organized, related systems of connections is simply by making use of the general law of association. If the pupil is to have facts together in useful systems, the teacher must put them together. If in the future the pupil is to think of the relations of a fact when he thinks of the fact, he must in the present connect that fact with those relations.

The commonest means of securing this connection between a fact and its relations is to teach them at the same time, *e. g.,* to teach the arithmetic of latitude and longitude in the same month in which the geography of latitude and longitude is taught. This is an excellent means, but it is not always the best and is often very hard

Principles of Association 129

to arrange without conflict with other desirable features of teaching. Thus it is not the best in the case of percentage and interest and cannot be arranged in the case of English grammar, Latin grammar and German grammar without overtaxing the capacity of high-school students.

Teaching the two things to be related at the same time is in fact not the essential in correlation, but only one means. The essential is that the two be related *in the pupil's mind.* One may be taught five years after the other, but if its relations with the other are then made a part of the pupil's mental equipment, all may be well. One may be taught by one teacher and the other by another teacher, but if each teacher makes the necessary cross-connections, the two systems of connections in the pupil's mind will henceforth cooperate.

The chief dangers to be avoided in teaching relationships are: (1) such an infatuation with the doctrine of correlation as leads one to waste time in teaching relationships so obvious that a pupil is sure to make them for himself or so trivial that they are not worth the making, and (2) such ignorance or carelessness as leads one to teach relationships that are false or artificial. It is as bad or even worse to teach a useless relationship as a useless fact, a false relationship as a false fact.

§ 33. *Exercises*

1. To what extent would you relate arithmetic and manual training?

2. To what extent would you relate arithmetic and elementary science?

3. To what extent would you relate English history and English literature (in the high school)?

9

130   *The Principles of Teaching*

4. To what extent would you relate the study of the Latin language and the study of Roman life?

5. To what extent would you relate English composition and chemistry (in the high school)?

6. Give two cases of important relationships (a) between the history of the United States and its geography. (b) Between the United States constitution and United States history. (c) Between drawing and other elementary-school subjects. (d) Between high-school mathematics and high-school science.

7. In which of the following cases should a teacher specially relate the two members of the pair? In which cases is it not worth while to do so?

> a. The Latin *civilis* and the English *civil*.
> b. The Latin *pecus* and *pecunia*.
> c. The German *Vaterland* and the English *fatherland*.
> d. Decimal fractions and the metric system.
> e. Addition or subtraction and the study of the crow.
> f. The growth of seeds and moral lessons on patience and persistence.
> g. The climate of Central America and the dress of its inhabitants.

8. In the case of each of the relationships not worth teaching state whether the cause is (a) that the relation is sure to be learned anyway or (b) that it is too trivial to spend time on or (c) that it is false.

9. (a) State a just objection to each one of the practices described below. (b) State also some compensating (or partially compensating) advantage of the practice, where such exists.

> a. Relating all the work of a class during December to the topic, Christmas.

Principles of Association   131

   b. Teaching pronunciation, definitions, usages of language, spelling and the like in connection with the reading of literature.

   c. Teaching composition in connection with literature, that is, having pupils write about the books they read.

   d. Correlating all the work in music with history, that is, teaching children to sing Indian songs when they are studying the settling of America; teaching them to sing hymns when they are studying the Pilgrim fathers, and the like.

   e. Putting words of one sort together in each spelling lesson as in the following[1]:—

"Rule—Nouns ending in Y with a vowel before it, form the plural by adding S without changing the Y; as Key, Keys.

Henry VIII. abolished abbies and convents. The viceroies were attended by countless lackies. The jockies could not manage the donkies. The larder displays turkies and geese. Criminals in France are confined in a sort of public vessels called gallies. The vallies are overflowed. The public monies are no where safe from peculation. It is the custom to fire several vollies over the grave of a soldier. The kidnies are among the lower viscera. Chimnies are seldom seen in hot climates. A king of England died of excess in eating lampries." [38]

"CH as K.

Tecknical words are those peculiar to the arts and sciences. He was placed in a new sepulcre. A chymera is a creature of the imagination. A hemistick is half a line of poetry. Mineral waters containing iron are called calibeate. The camelion is a reptile of the lizard genus. The first point in chyrography or penmanship, should be distinctness. Concology treats of shells. Any instrument that measures time is a cronometer. An anacronism is the placing of an event at a wrong date. Sinecdoche is a figure of speech." [39]

[1] These lessons are designed, of course, to teach the pupil spelling by having him correct the misspellings.

132 *The Principles of Teaching*

 f. Relating spelling to object lessons as suggested
  by this quotation:

'Lessons in spelling may frequently be made from objects, by taking the name of an object, the names of its parts, words denoting the uses of the object, and other words suggested by the object or associated with it.' [40]

For Further Reading

 W. James, *Talks to Teachers on Psychology*, Chapters VIII, IX and XII.

 J. Adams, *Herbartian Psychology Applied to Education*, Chapter VII.

CHAPTER IX

THE PRINCIPLES OF ANALYSIS

Preparatory, *Elements of Psychology*, §§ 38-40

§ 34. *Principles of Teaching*

The mind's most frequent intellectual act is to connect one thing with another, but its highest performance is to think a thing apart into its elements. Dissociation or analysis furnishes the data for the advanced types of human thinking and action and, by giving a chance for the operation of the law of partial activity, is the basis of reasoning and intelligent morality. For the habits of human thought are not merely habits of response to the actual gross situations of life, to 'being hungry when in sight of an apple tree' or 'being sleepy in bed' or 'being struck by a foe,' but are responses to whole classes of situations at once and to detailed elements, aspects and features of situation. We can respond to the quality eight, regardless of whether it be eight kittens, eight dollars, eight elephants or eight trees,—to the quality round, regardless of whether it be the ring of a circus or the ring of a bride.

To teach the meaning of *six* or *unless* or *because* to a primary class, the laws of mood and tense to students beginning the study of grammar, the principles of the order of the sentence in German,—in all cases where the facts to be appreciated or the laws to be understood con-

133

134 *The Principles of Teaching*

cern something beyond direct experiences of concrete things and events,—something more is needed than putting one thing with another in the way they ought to go. One thing must be put *with many things, with some one feature of which it is to go.* Stimuli must now be so arranged that certain elements or aspects hitherto undefined or even unexperienced will be clearly felt, that certain general and abstract judgments will emerge from the given facts.

This same power of analysis is involved in teaching the more advanced, abstract and general facts from the starting-point of simpler abstractions already learned. Knowledge of the meaning of 'a number' is gained from knowledge of the meaning of two, six, eight, thirteen, twenty, one-half and six-tenths, just as the knowledge of the meaning of 'six' is gained from experience of six blocks, six balls, six books, six trees, and the like. The meaning of virtue comes similarly from already acquired meanings of bravery, sympathy, honesty and the like.

The same process of analysis is involved in those subtler forms of reasoning which we call judgment, tact and intuition as well as in reasoning outright. Many experiences of faces, differing in features, complexion, etc., but alike in some subtle signs of dishonesty, produce in the trained judge of men the judgment, 'a lack of straightforwardness,' about any individual of that general type. Many experiences of the weather, alike in some subtle and undescribed combination of wind, cloudiness, etc., and different in all else, develop the connection between the judgment, 'It will rain,' and any day of a certain type.

Whenever, in fact, the intellect responds to a part or aspect which it experiences only in complex mixtures, whether by explicit thought or by subtle intuition, its

The Principles of Analysis 135

response depends on the law of analysis. In teaching, therefore, whenever the desired response concerns an element or aspect experienced only in complex mixtures, the principle will be to provide the conditions which favor the operation of the law of analysis. These are:—

1. Experiences of enough total facts, in each of which (a) the element is as obtrusive as possible, as little encumbered by irrelevant detail as possible, and in which (b) the element's concomitants or surroundings vary.

. 2. The comparison of these facts with attention directed toward the elements or parts of each fact, especially toward the element in question.

3. The association of a convenient verbal description of the element with it through association with each of its manifestations. (The convenient verbal description is commonly twofold, a definition which describes the element well and a name or symbol which is brief and refers to it without ambiguity. Thus we have 'Density is the ratio of the mass to the volume of a body' and the symbol 'D.')

4. Repeated practice in responding correctly to the element in new complexes.

§ 35. *Their Application: Exercises*

1. What was the probable defect in the instruction which led to this incident? A child was being displayed by his fond parents. Says the father, holding a knife in a vertical position, 'What do you call that?' 'I calls it a knife.' 'Yes, it is a knife, but think what you learned the other day at kindergarten.' 'I calls it a knife.' No coaxing succeeds in eliciting anything but knife, till the mother tries with a pencil held upright. To this the desired response comes, 'I calls it vertical.' [41]

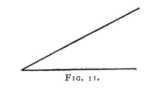

FIG. 11.

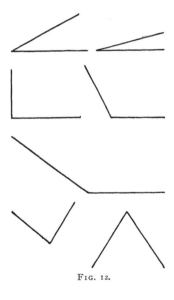

FIG. 12.

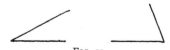

FIG. 13.

2. Why do children not learn from their general experience of words that to express the fact that something is done to a person or thing some word like *is, was, are,* or *be* is used with another word telling what the 'something done' is?

3. In teaching the definition of an angle at the beginning of high-school geometry, which figure is the better, one like FIG. 11 or one like FIG. 12? Why?

4. Which would show the essential fact, the difference in direction between two lines, least encumbered with the irrelevant detail of the length to which the lines are extended, FIG. 13 or FIG. 14?

5. What is the value of such an exercise as:— Name all the angles in FIG. 15?

6. Of this:—Name ten angles in FIG. 16.

7. Of this:—Name five pairs of lines in FIG. 16 such that in each pair there is no difference of direction.

The Principles of Analysis

8. Which of the following cases of the use of *although* is the better fitted to give knowledge of its meaning, (A) or (B)?

9. Give the reason for your choice.

A. Although he is a farmer, he is very rich.
Although it was Sunday, he went outdoors.

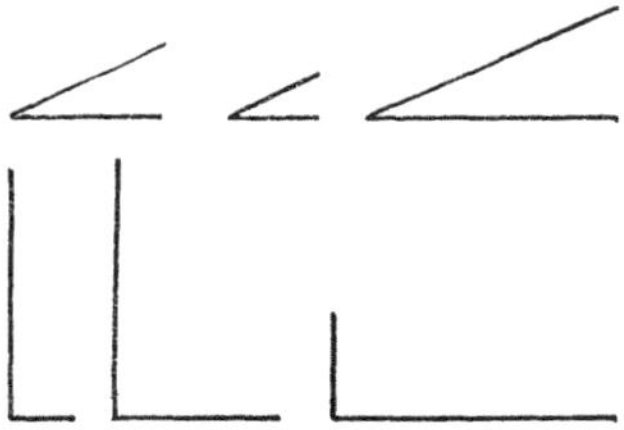

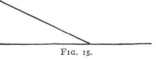
Fig. 14.

B. Although he is awake, his eyes are shut.
Although it was Monday, there was no school.

10. Give four or five other sentences varying the concomitants of *although,* and so chosen as to attract attention to its meaning.

11. What would be the effect of giving the class at the same time these sentences?

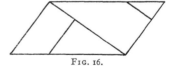
Fig. 15.

Because he is awake, his eyes are open.
Because it is Monday, there will probably be school.

12. Which of the following exercises in application of the knowledge is the better, (A) or (B)? Why?

A.
Put in each empty space the word

Fig. 16.

although if it makes a sensible or true statement out of the sentence and the word *because* if it makes a sensible or true statement out of the sentence. Put in the word that makes the sentence sound best.

138 *The Principles of Teaching*

Four three's are twelve   if you add
three and three and three and three you get
twelve.

       four three's are twelve, four twenty-
three's are not twenty twelve.

I will not eat   I would like to.

He plays   he likes to.

He knew it was ten o'clock   he heard
the bell.

They are very big   they are very young.

They are very small   they are sixteen
years old.

She runs   she is tired.

B.

Write two sentences with *although* in each.

Tell me something, using the word *although*.

13. Underline once those of the questions and directions below which are designed to give experiences of enough total facts in which the concomitants of the element, difference in direction of two lines, vary.

14. Underline twice those which are designed to make the element as obtrusive as possible and as little encumbered by irrelevant detail as possible.

15. In what way in these questions and exercises is attention directed toward the element, difference in direction?

Take pencil, paper and a ruler. Make five points on the sheet an inch or so apart. Mark them P^1, P^2, P^3, etc. From point 1 draw a line in a horizontal direction and to the right. Mark it line 1. Draw another line from point 1 in a vertical direction toward the top of the paper. Mark it line 2. Draw from point 2 a line to the right as you did before but twice as long. Mark it line 3.

The Principles of Analysis 139

Draw from point 2 a line in a vertical direction as you did line 2 but twice as long. Mark it line 4. From point 3 draw two lines with a difference in direction half that between lines 1 and 2. Mark them line 5 and line 6. From point 4 draw two lines with a difference in direction one and a half times that between line 1 and line 2. Mark the lines line 7 and line 8. We may name any angle by naming its sides and point or vertex. Thus the first angle we drew would be called angle 1 P^1 2, the one we drew next would be called angle 3 P^2 4. Draw from point 5 lines 9 and 10 making an angle,—that is, a difference in direction,—equal to angle 5 P^3 6, but make the lines only half as long as lines 5 and 6. Cover part of the lines 7 and 8. Is the angle 7 P^4 8 any smaller? What angle drawn is equal to angle 1 P^1 2?

Take two threads both tied at one end to the same thumb-tack and each tied at the other end to a separate pin. Fasten the thumb-tack in the middle of one cover of your note-book. Stretch out one thread and stick the pin firmly in the cover. Now stretch out the other thread so that it lies just on top of the first thread, having the same direction. Do the two threads make an angle? None or, we might say, a zero angle, since their difference in direction is zero. Swing the unfastened pin around till it makes with the fixed thread an angle equal to 5 P^3 6. Swing it further till the angle is equal to 1 P^1 2. Swing it further till it is just in line with the fixed thread but extending in the opposite direction. The difference in direction between the two parts of a straight line turned the one in the opposite direction from the other is called a straight angle. Move the thread still further. If we count the angle or difference in direction along the path that the thread has followed, the angle is greater than a straight angle. Such an angle is called

140   *The Principles of Teaching*

a reflex angle. Swing the thread still further until it is nearly back to its starting place. The difference in direction or angle between it and the fixed thread is now almost equal to two straight angles if we count the difference in direction along the path the thread has followed, and almost equal to zero if we count it along the unfollowed path toward the original position.

How many straight angles would the difference in direction between north and south be? To what direction would $1\frac{1}{2}$ straight angles bring you, starting from north and turning toward the west? To what direction would 2 straight angles bring you, starting from due east?

16. What total facts would you select as the material by considering which a pupil could come to know the abstract element, 'a negative quantity'?

17. Answer the same question in the case of the meaning of 'a noun.'

18. In the case of the meaning of 'unless.'

19. In the case of the meaning of 'one-sixth.'

20. In the case of the meaning of 'wealth.'

21. In the case of the law of the result of the combination of an acid and a base.

22. In the case of the meaning of 'acceleration.'

23. State in three or more of these cases how you would make sure that the attention of the student was directed toward the essential element.

24. In which one of the seven cases is a useful definition most difficult?

25. What is the advantage of such a name for an angle as $\angle$? Of $A+B=H+S$ in place of 'an acid combined with a base gives hydrogen and a salt'?

26. Make out for two or more of the seven cases ten exercises each in detecting the element in new complexes.

The Principles of Analysis 141

27. What words would you select for phonic drill on at (as in hat), ate (as in mate), ick (as in stick) and ike (as in strike)?

In many cases a pupil's previous experience has provided enough total facts presenting the element or aspect in question with varying concomitants, but the process of analysis has not been made, or has been made only partially or crudely, or has resulted in the abstraction of some insignificant or non-essential feature. So with *blue* for some kindergarten children, *square* for primary school children, *river* for those in the fourth grade, *weight* for those in the eighth, *density* and *heat* for high-school pupils. In such cases the work of teaching is to direct attention to the facts already known or to extend, refine or replace the previous work of analysis.

28. Is the task of teaching the difference between a mechanical mixture and a chemical compound in the first year of high school chiefly to provide certain total facts or to call attention to certain aspects of facts already often experienced?

29. What additional facts would you provide to extend the work of previous analysis in the case of teaching the definition of weight to high-school pupils? Choose from the following list:

a. Air has weight.
b. The gas in a balloon has weight.
c. A chair has weight.
d. A feather has weight.
e. The moon has weight.
f. Ambition has not weight.
g. Love has not weight.
h. An apple has weight.
i. The weight of a quart of water or of a cubic

142 *The Principles of Teaching*

inch of lead or of your hat is not the same on the top of a mountain as in a valley below.

j. A headache has not weight.

k. The desire to eat candy has not weight.

30. Before reading the next paragraphs write out a definition of heat. Write out also a definition of temperature. Then study the paragraphs. Note the changes which they make in your ideas of these two facts and the means by which they make them. Note especially what previous experiences are selected for review, what new experience is given, what use is made of comparison, what use is made of contrast, and how care is taken that the student learns facts rather than words.

I. DISTINCTION BETWEEN HEAT AND TEMPERATURE

"218. Most people will agree that a cup of water taken from a boiling kettle has, at the instant it is dipped out, the same temperature as that of the boiling water. Most people will likewise agree that for heating purposes the large kettle is much more efficient than the small cup of water. A water bag or a water bottle that holds a gallon will give out more heat and give it out longer, other things being equal, than one which holds only a pint. If the temperatures of the two vessels of water are the same, the larger is said to contain more heat. If a bath tub be half filled with cold water, one can heat it more by pouring in a gallon of boiling water than by putting in a quart of boiling water; for, although the temperatures are the same, the gallon contains more heat than the quart. These simple facts are cited merely to show that popular notions concerning the distinction between heat and temperature are perfectly clear. They are also correct. But before the word temperature can be admitted to the rather select vocabulary of physics, it must be defined in unmistakable English. This we now proceed to do.

Imagine three vessels of water, A, B, C (Fig. 110), (FIG. 17 here) each containing a different quantity of water. If A and B are placed side by side, in contact, and B thereby gains heat,—be it ever so little,—A has imparted heat to B; and A is said to have a higher temperature than B.

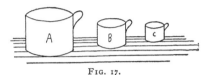

FIG. 17.

Put C in contact with B; if B thereby loses heat,—be it ever so little,—heat has passed into C; and C is said to be at a lower temperature than B.

When, in general, one body is placed in contact with another, the difference of temperature between the bodies is that which determines which way the heat flows. If the heat flows from A to B, A has the higher temperature; but if the heat flows from B to A, then B has the higher temperature.

Consider two vessels of water, E and F (Fig. 111), (Fig. 18 here) connected by a rubber tube. Does the

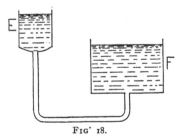

FIG· 18.

water always flow from the large vessel to the small one? What does determine the direction of the flow? If the water flows from E to F, does the surface of the water in F rise by the same amount that the surface in E falls?

144   *The Principles of Teaching*

Returning now to Fig. 110, heat the water in the smaller vessel C, nearly to the boiling point, while the water in A has about the temperature of the room. Place a thermometer in each vessel, and then put the vessel C into A, without allowing the liquids to mix. Does the temperature of C fall as much as that of A rises?

Point out clearly the analogy between temperature and level; also between change of temperature and change of level.

219. The following definitions will now be clear to everyone who has mastered the foregoing facts:

"Definition of Temperature.—*The temperature of a body is its thermal state considered with reference to its power of communicating heat to other bodies.*

"Definition of Higher and Lower Temperature.— *If when two bodies are placed in thermal communication, one of the bodies loses heat, and the other gains heat, that body which gives out heat is said to have a higher temperature than that which receives heat from it.*

"Corollary.—*If when two bodies are placed in thermal communication neither of them loses or gains heat, the two bodies are said to have equal temperatures or the same temperature. The two bodies are then said to be in thermal equilibrium.*

"Law of Equal Temperatures.—*Bodies whose temperatures are equal to that of the same body have themselves equal temperatures.*"—Maxwell, *Theory of Heat,* Ch. II.

The point in this definition which calls for emphasis is the fact that temperature is a state of a body. 'It is a condition which confronts us.'" [42]

31. Plan a lesson the aim of which shall be to refine the inadequate idea of the likenesses and differences between animals and plants possessed by beginners in biology.

32. The qualities of a good description of an abstracted element, in other words of a good definition of the word which names it, are precision and simplicity. "To be precise is to tell exactly what the word means—

The Principles of Analysis 145

no more and no less; to state the characteristics of an object, in virtue of which the name is applicable, with perfect definiteness. To be simple in a definition is to frame it in such a way that it will immediately mean something to the people for whom it is intended." [43]

Score each of the following definitions as good or poor in precision (gp or pp) and also as good or poor in simplicity (gs or ps).

a. Addition is the putting together of two or more numbers so as to make but one. [44]

b. Arithmetical progression is when a series of numbers increases by a common excess, or decreases by a common difference. [45]

c. The inclination of two lines meeting one another, or the opening between them, is called an angle. [46]

d. The process of finding the difference between two numbers is called subtraction. [47]

e. The product of several equal factors is called a power of one of them. [48]

f. To multiply a number (the multiplicand) by an abstract number (the multiplier) is to do to the former what is done to unity to obtain the latter. [49]

g. Velocity is......the time rate of change of position of the particle. [50]

h. The velocity of a motion is the space traversed in a unit of time. It may be in miles per hour, feet per second, etc. [51]

i. Density is simply the ratio of the mass to the volume of a body. $D = \dfrac{M}{V}$ [52]

j. The density of a substance is the amount of matter in a given bulk. It is determined by the weight of the substance. A cubic inch of lead is heavier than a cubic inch of wood because it is more dense. Density is entirely distinct from hardness. [53]

146 *The Principles of Teaching*

k. An adjective is a word joined by way of description or limitation to a noun or a pronoun. [54]

l. A noun is a word used as a name. [55]

m. A noun is the name of a thing.

n. A verb is the name of an action.

For Further Reading

C. A. McMurry and F. M. McMurry, *The Method of the Recitation,* Chapter II.

CHAPTER X

REASONING

Preparatory, *Elements of Psychology*, §§ 48 and 49

§ 36. *Reasoning as Selective Thinking*

General Principles.—The processes of judging facts, reasoning, following an argument and reaching conclusions are the same processes of association and dissociation as are found in all learning; the difference is that there is active selection within the present thought of some part or aspect · which consequently determines the next thought, and selection again amongst the sequent thoughts, retaining one and discarding others. The laws of rational thought are, that is, the general laws of association and dissociation, but with predominance of the law of partial activity. The principles of teaching in the case of responses of comprehension, inference, invention and the like are the principles of apperception, habit formation and analysis, but special importance now attaches to principles derived from the fact that (1) the total set or context or system of thought and (2) any single feature of a thought, as well as the particular thing thought of, may decide the future course of thinking.

The principles thus derived are: (1) Arouse in the pupil's mind the system of ideas and connections relevant to the work in hand. (2) Lead him to examine each

148   *The Principles of Teaching*

fact he thinks of in the light of the aim of that work and to focus attention on the element of the fact which is essential to his aim. (3) Insist that he test whether or not it is the essential by making sure that it leads on to the goal aimed at and by the logical step of verification, by comparing the conclusions to which it leads with known facts.

Thus in helping a class to reason out the answer to the problem, 'Why is it wise for people suffering from consumption to go to Denver rather than stay in New York City?', a teacher would ask such suggestive questions as: 'What do you know about the causes and cure of consumption? What are some features of location which influence health? What are some other differences between New York and Denver which are important from the point of view of health?' Unless a pupil's trains of thought lay within the general system of 'thoughts of physical and social forces of cities which act on health,' there would be little chance of his reasoning well. Supposing that latitude, longitude, altitude, nature of prevailing winds, size of the cities, differences in the occupations of their inhabitants, mountains *versus* level country, well-water *versus* tap-water and other facts have been offered as explanations, good teaching will (2) encourage the pupil to attend to each of these facts from the point of view of the difference to a consumptive. What difference in latitude is there between New York and Denver? How would latitude in itself influence climate? Davos, Switzerland, the Adirondack Mountains and Ashville, N. C., are all noted resorts for consumptives. How much influence has latitude? Does longitude make the difference? Why not? In what respects are Denver, Ashville, Davos and other resorts for consumptives alike? What are some features of

Reasoning 149

climate that are specially injurious to consumptives? Finally when the pupil concludes that, say, the greater evenness of temperature throughout the year leads consumptives to prefer Denver, the teacher will require him to show that in point of fact less variability in temperature does exist there, and that it is favorable to consumptives.

The three principles may be illustrated further in connection with the following problem :—

A pays $10,000 for a bond, 4 per cent. interest on which is paid every Dec. 31 for 10 years, at the end of which the $10,000 principal is paid. On the same date B pays $10,000 for a farm, for the rent of which he receives every Dec. 31 for 10 years 10 per cent. of the farm's assessed valuation, which at the time of purchase is $5,000. On Dec. 31 of each year B pays in taxes 2 per cent. of the assessed valuation. Each year his farm increases in value $200. Who made the better investment, A or B?

(1) The arousal of relevant systems of arithmetical knowledge and ideas of profit and loss is almost certainly a result of the statement of the problem itself. The teacher may have to assist the pupil, however, (2) to 'focus attention on the element of the fact which is essential.' Thus it will be advantageous for the pupil to arrange the facts as (A) amounts of income and principal due to owning the bond and (B) amounts of income and principal due to owning the real estate. It will also help in the solution of the problem if the pupil observes that the initial cost is the same and that the essential is therefore the amount in hand at the end of each year. It will also help the pupil if, after finding that in the first year the real estate bargain has netted an equal income and a rise in value of $200, he thinks of the facts that by the conditions of the problem the rent of the real

150 *The Principles of Teaching*

estate will thereafter exceed the interest on the bond and that the rise in value continues.

The step of verification by actual fact, that is by finding two such properties, buying them and counting the profits after ten years, is of course unnecessary as well as impracticable here.

Difficulties in Teaching Reasoning.—There is no royal road to teaching subjects requiring reasoning. The student must have the facts to reason with and have them arranged in systems in the way in which they will be needed. He must replace the gross total fact which suggests nothing or a thousand irrelevant things by that one of its elements or features or aspects that does suggest some consequence of use for the solution of the problem in hand. He must learn to criticise his ideas so as to know which do show signs of usefulness for his purpose, when to give a line of thought up as hopeless, and what he has proved when he has finished. He must make sure that he has not somewhere made a slip by testing his conclusion by actual experience or by comparison with facts absolutely certain.

The teacher's work in guiding rational thought bears much the same relation to his work in habit formation that teaching a child to himself find the way to go from his house to one a mile away would bear to teaching him to follow the road there. In the latter case you have only to put certain acts with certain situations,—going to the right by the mill, taking the path at the top of the ridge and the like. But in the former you must make sure that the youngster knows what place he is to try to reach and keeps it in mind. He must also at least know that to get to a place you must keep going and not lie down to sleep; he must have some knowledge of the direction in which the house lies and of the roads and

Reasoning 151

woods and valley in the neighborhood. He starts off correctly and at a cross-road turns to the left. 'What did you do that for, John?' 'I don't know.' 'Where are you going?' 'To grandpa's.' 'Where does that road go?' 'To the school-house.' 'Is that on the way to grandpa's?' 'I don't know.' 'What comes after the school-house if you go down this road?' 'The church.' 'How long does it take to go from grandpa's to the church?' 'Oh! a long time.' 'Is grandpa's near the church?' 'No. It is a long way.' 'This road goes to the church. Is it a good way to go to grandpa's?'

If your boy is bright enough, he now turns to the right, but soon comes to the end of the road. 'Where do I go now?' says he. 'Where do you think?' 'I think we go through that field.' 'Well, try it and see!' You rapidly approach a pond and the boy sits down and cries. 'I can't find the way to grandpa's.' 'What's the trouble?' 'You can't get around this pond, it's all swampy.' 'Do you have to go around it?' 'Yes. Grandpa's is up there and you have to go around the pond.' 'Go and look at the pond and see if you can find anything about it that will help you to get to grandpa's.' And so on with constant stimulation to the examination of each situation confronted and with the selection and rejection of ways in the light of knowledge of their consequences, until grandpa's house is reached, or until the problem in arithmetic is solved.

The Use of Comparison, Contrast and Analysis.— The teacher's chief means to aid the pupil in holding his mind to the point at issue, analyzing facts into their elements, choosing the right element and testing progress by results, are (provided the facts needed to reason with are surely possessed) *comparison, contrast* and *analysis*.

For instance, suppose that the teacher's problem is to

152 *The Principles of Teaching*

make a pupil really understand that in international trade the country which has a money balance owed to it as the result of the year's trade is not necessarily the gainer. The following somewhat crude lesson will show clearly the value of comparison and contrast:—

You have 100 horses of equal value and are dealing with three men, Jones, Smith and Brown, each of whom has 100 cows, all 300 being of equal value. In trade with Jones you give 10 horses for 20 cows. In the trade with Smith you give 10 horses for 10 cows and 100 dollars. In trade with Brown you give 10 horses for 105 dollars. In which case do you have the largest money balance? Is the trade with Brown the most advantageous of the three?

Make a statement of your trade with Jones, Smith and Brown, *e. g.,*

	Gave	*Received*
J.	10 horses.	20 cows.
S.	10 horses.	10 cows and 100 dollars.
B.	10 horses.	105 dollars.

Suppose that you trade as before with Jones, Smith and Brown and sell a fourth man, Adams, 10 of the 20 cows you get from Jones, receiving from him 10 horses of equal value with your first 100? In trading with Jones and Adams do you have any money balance? Do you make any real profit? Make a statement of your trade with Jones and Adams, with Smith and with Brown.

Suppose that you trade as before but instead of selling Smith 10 horses for 10 cows and 100 dollars, you sold him 10 horses for 100 dollars. Is your money balance from the trade any less? Is your gain any less?

The following cases will show the value of analysis of the fact, balance of trade, into its elements:

Reasoning 153

Suppose that your nation has ten horses, a thousand dollars, ten cows, two houses, six chairs, two suits of clothes and provisions for a year.

Suppose that the only other nations of the world are A, B and C, which have each the same amount of property and of money as your nation.

If after a year of trade A, B and C had each $1333\frac{1}{3}$ dollars and your nation had all of their property, which would be the best off?

Would the case be different if the figures were 1333333 dollars, provided your nation had acquired *all* of the property?

Which does an individual or a nation desire in the long run, more things or more money?

If nation A exports to nation B and nation C the same quantities of products and gets in return from nation B 1000 bales of silk and 2000 dollars, and from nation C 1000 bales of the same silk and 200 automobiles, what decides which trade is the more advantageous?

Limitations to Teaching.—Constant control, consideration of possibilities, recall of the consequences of each possibility, testing, trying another, proving its fitness, searching for the next step in view of the end to be reached and the like make rational thinking more difficult for the pupil and its direction more difficult for the teacher than is the case with simple habit formation.

Moreover the capacity to think in parts and to think things together comes later in life and is weaker than the capacity to put one thing with another. Nature limits teaching more sharply in the logic of arithmetic than in its computation; in the theory of language than in its use; in the appreciation of scientific arguments than in simply knowing scientific facts. There are by nature many more learners than thinkers. Teaching must not

154   *The Principles of Teaching*

be blamed for not doing what only natural gifts can do.

What teaching can do is to see that the aim of the work is known, that the facts to reason with are known, and that they are arranged in useful systems; to check the pupil in his pursuit of irrelevant ideas, helping him early or late in each such side-excursion to see that he is off the track; to bring into relief the elements of any fact by comparison, contrast and analysis; to suggest ways of testing the validity of each step; and to develop the habits of deliberation, criticism and verification. In the case of two special forms of thought, somewhat more definite principles of guidance can be given. These will be postponed to separate sections on *Inductive Teaching* and *Deductive Teaching*.

SUMMARY

So-called Reasoning is the result of ordinary habits of thought plus selection. Good teaching provides the basis for this selective thinking, knowledge of the goal to reason toward and of the facts to reason with, arouses and guides it by the help of comparison, contrast and analysis and forms the habit of always verifying its results.

§ 37. *Inductive Methods of Teaching*

Induction and Deduction.—In the common meaning of the words, inductive thinking is inference that progresses from particular facts to a general conclusion or from a series of general facts to a still more general conclusion, while deductive thinking is inference from a general fact to some particular fact or from a more general fact to some less general fact. There are many objec-

Reasoning 155

tions to these definitions from the point of view of psychology and also from that of logic, but for the purpose of making a distinction between two common processes in teaching, they are unobjectionable.

Following this common usage, inductive teaching may be defined as teaching some general fact on the basis of knowledge of particular or of less general facts; deductive teaching, as teaching some fact on the basis of knowledge of a more general fact. Experimental work in science, in which particular facts are acquired, grouped, compared and made to suggest a general law, is the type of inductive teaching; geometry, in which from a few axioms about equals and unequals and a few simple premises in the shape of definitions of lines, angles, and the like, the student is shown how to prove some other general truth, is the type of the latter.

In the actual thinking of the class-room, inductions and deductions are intermingled each with the other and both with inferences from one particular to another particular and from one general to another of the same degree of generality. It is, however, convenient to treat the two methods of teaching separately.

Direct and Analytic Inductions.—Facts to be taught inductively are of two sorts: (1) Cases where the general fact is simply the uniform occurrence of some connection between two gross, concrete, easily observed facts; *e. g.,* that every day is followed by a night, that if you put your finger in a flame it feels hot, that if you let go of an apple it falls. (2) Cases where the general fact is the uniform occurrence of some connection between two facts one of which (or both of which) is a partial or abstract fact which can be thought about only after it has been analyzed out of the complexes in which it inheres; *e. g.,* that oxygen causes rust, that the moon is

156 *The Principles of Teaching*

the cause of the tides, that bacilli which produce lactic acid are the cause of the souring of milk. These two classes of facts are not, however, sharply separated; there is a gradation from the most obvious to the most abstract.

Principles of Teaching.—The teaching of inductions of the first sort is essentially the formation of a mental habit and the principle to be followed is that of habit formation. The teaching of the second sort is essentially the abstraction of an element plus the formation of a mental habit. The principles of teaching here grow directly out of the principles of analysis, the essentials of method being (1) *a clear statement of the goal aimed at,* (2) *the selection of enough and representative individual facts,* (3) *their arrangement in such a way as to make the general idea or judgment to which they lead obvious,* (4) *the verification of the conclusion by an appeal to known facts,* and (5) *its reinforcement and clarification by exercises in applying it to new individual facts.*

In practice, a teacher must often, indeed usually, sacrifice the advantages of 'enough' facts to economize time. If the data really desirable as a basis for teaching inductively the influence of a hot climate on the activities of man were presented, a score of lesson periods would be required. It becomes all the more necessary to choose representative facts, facts that are a fair sampling of the whole class to be considered. Thus in teaching about rivers, the Mississippi, Tennessee and Connecticut would be a better three than the Potomac, Hudson and Connecticut since the latter are all of the peculiar estuary variety.

The crucial point in inductive teaching is the arrangement of the individual facts so as to make the general idea or judgment to which they lead obvious. For this the utmost ingenuity in using comparison and contrast is

Reasoning

often necessary. The pupil must be led to think in parts or elements and to select the right part or element. The principles to follow are the principles of selective attention and analysis.

The verification of conclusions is the keystone of correct inductive thinking in the world at large and should be more prominent in the school. The common practice of children is to accept as true whatever the teacher does not oppose. This is not so bad as it may seem, for 'to be accepted by the expert' is a sort of verification well known and not despised by science, and to the scholar the teacher stands *'in loco experti.'* Verification by actual experiment or observation is, however, preferable as a matter of training; and recourse to other authorities than the teacher provides useful experience of the bulk of expert knowledge which is stored up in dictionaries, encyclopaedias, tables, maps, books, and the like.

In such a case as learning from experiments with or discussions of the facts, 'friction causing heat,' 'impact of falling bodies causing heat,' 'an electric current causing heat' and the like, that heat is a mode of energy, the pupil's reasoning is imperfect until he does at least something in the way of experimental verification, such, for instance, as repeating Joule's experiment of expending given quantities of energy in raising the temperature of a vessel of water by friction. In such a case as learning inductively from experiments or discussions the fact of erosion, a pupil's reasoning is not complete until he has not only prophesied but also verified the result of making a brook go down a certain valley, or of leaving a mound of dirt exposed to a heavy shower. The best answer a pupil can make to the question, 'How do you know that the Hudson river carries soil from one place to another?', is to bring

158 *The Principles of Teaching*

you a bottle of water from the river and show you the sediment in it.

The Use of Types.—Many of the advantages of inductive teaching can be secured through a compromise between an out and out induction and a mere statement of conclusions, namely, through the type method. The thorough study of one typical case of a class or law gives a basis of real experience which serves to interpret, though not to prove, the general statement. Knowledge about such a type also serves as a center of attraction for later knowledge of things like it.

If a class in physical geography has but two weeks to give to the study of rivers, it will probably be best to give half of the time to one river alone, say the Mississippi. Since it is out of the question to teach the characteristics of the mammals by a valid induction, the choice is left between a very superficial study of many, an inadequate study of four or five or a thorough study of one form, for instance the rabbit, alone.

Thus one of the best of recent text-books on zoology (Parker and Haswell's) bases its discussion of each topic upon a thorough study of some one selected type. In the case of the birds, for instance, the arrangement of the section is as follows:

An introduction of less than half a page stating the most general features of the Class.

1. Example of the Class. The Common Pigeon (Columbia livia). This type study occupies 30 pages.

2. Distinctive Character and Classification. 9 pages.

3. General Organization. 28 pages.

The same method is illustrated by teaching the syntax of a foreign language by model sentences, each serving as a type of some principle of grammar. Eysenbach's German grammar is a familiar example.

Reasoning

The loss in using types in place of an adequate survey of particulars is due to the decrease in actual inference on the part of pupils and the risk of appealing to mere memory. The special advantage of the use of types is economy of time and hence the possibility of presenting a richer and more varied content of knowledge in a subject as a whole.

The Formal Steps of Instruction.—The principles of inductive teaching have been formulated under the name of the *steps of instruction* or the *formal steps.* These are generally taken to be the following five:—

1. *Preparation:* A statement of the aim of the work and a recall of facts already known in the light of which the new facts will be appreciated. This step refers to the use of the principle of apperception in teaching.

2. *Presentation:* The knowledge of the 'enough and representative particular facts' is secured.

3. *Comparison and Abstraction:* By studying the particular facts presented the student derives the essential general fact or law.

4. *Generalization:* This general fact or law is expressed clearly by the pupil.

5. *Application:* New individual facts are judged by the aid of it.

As has been shown, the vital features of inductive teaching concern steps 2 and 3, the selection of the most instructive particulars and their treatment so as to secure the abstraction of the general fact or law. It is, in fact, only in step 3 that inductive reasoning is demanded of the pupil.

These five formal steps serve as a convenient aid to thought in planning one's inductive teaching, but a new step should be added between the fourth and fifth, namely a step of *verification,* in which the general conclusion is

160 *The Principles of Teaching*

tested by an appeal to facts. It should also be borne in mind that step 1 concerns the general principle of apperception rather than inductive teaching in particular, that step 4, though important, is brief and usually comes almost of itself once step 3 is successfully carried through, and that step 5 is deductive.

Unfortunately very much of so-called inductive teaching prolongs steps 1 and 2, heaping up in the latter particular facts unfairly selected, and then *makes step 3 for the pupil*, and leaves its result unverified.

Such teaching is as likely to form bad habits of thought as good, and if the pupil does gain real knowledge of the general truth, it is not by deriving it in step 3, but in the course of trying to apply it. To state a fact or law outright with a few well chosen illustrations is better teaching than to give such make-believe inductions.

§ 38. *Deductive Methods of Teaching*

Principles of Teaching.—Good teaching by deductive methods depends upon *a clear statement of the goal aimed at, independent search by pupils for the proper class under which to think of the fact in question, criticism by them and by the teacher of the different classes suggested,* and *appreciation of the reasons why the right one is the right one.*

The Causes of Difficulty in Deductive Thinking.— Deductive reasonings may be very easy or very hard to make. 'Shall I call *brevity* in the sentence, *Brevity is the soul of wit,* a noun or not?' is easy for any scholar who knows a little grammar. To prove that *if the bisectors of two angles of a triangle are equal, the angle is isosceles* by a direct demonstration based on no truths

Reasoning 161

other than those established in, say, Book I of Wentworth's Geometry, is extremely hard.

They are easy in proportion as the number of possible classes under which to think of the fact in question are known and are few, and in proportion as the consequences of being in each of such classes are known. Thus *brevity* can be only *a noun* or *not a noun*, and to decide that it is not a noun one needs only to decide that it is a noun or that it is not a verb, adjective, article, etc. How to translate *arma* in *Arma virumque cano Troiae qui primus ab oris,* etc., is easy because *arma* can only be nominative, accusative or vocative plural of *armum* or an imperative of *armare* and because the consequences of being nominative plural, being vocative plural, etc., are well known.

Deductive reasonings are hard in proportion as the possible classes under which to think of the given fact are unknown or numerous, and in proportion as the consequences of being in each of such are unknown. To give a direct proof of the proposition that if the bisectors of two angles of a triangle are equal the triangle is isosceles is hard because there are hundreds of ways of thinking of (or classes under which to subsume) a triangle with the bisectors of two of its angles equal, many of which the student will never have thought of at all. 'How to best legislate so as to decrease divorces?' is harder to answer than, 'How to translate *arma?*' because the law to decrease divorce is a thing of such varied possibilities and also because the consequences of each one of these are so little known.

The Search for the Essential Quality.—The crucial step in deductive teaching is the direction of the pupil's search for the proper class under which to think of the fact in question. This implies picking out the element or aspect of the fact in question which is essential for the

162 *The Principles of Teaching*

problem in hand. Can you farm profitably on the banks of the Nile? Think of the Nile as a river with such and such a river basin and as a river with an annual overflow. 'How shall you bridge the Nile?' Think of the Nile as so wide and deep and with such and such a bottom. 'How far can you sail up the Nile?' Think of the Nile as so deep, with such and such falls and cataracts. 'Shall a town pump its drinking water from the Nile?' Think of the Nile above the town only and of its sources of contamination. So long as one thought of the Nile only as in the class 'wide rivers' or as in the class 'typhoid-bearing' rivers, he would be unable to deduce anything about the fertility of its banks.

Because of the difficulty of this step, all save a very few text-books omit it and tell the pupil what the element essential to his purpose is in the case of all but the very easy deductions. In geometry, for instance, the proofs are for the most part given; in arithmetic examples of a certain sort are given in direct connection with the principle under which they come; in geography questions are asked in a context which gives direct clues to the class under which the scholar must think of the fact to get the right answer. For instance, the question, 'Why do so few plants grow in a desert?' hardly requires any independent search by the pupil who meets the question immediately after having read: 'A desert has scarcely any rain. Here and there is a small extent of country where the ground is moistened by water from springs. In such places the soil is fertile and is covered with plants.'

The essential step in reasoning must sometimes be omitted in order to preserve the less capable pupils from vain efforts or random guessing and to save time. But the wise course is not to eliminate altogether the inde-

Reasoning

pendent search by pupils for the proper class, but to make it easier and briefer by directing it.

It is made easier (1) by systematizing the process of search, (2) by limiting the number of classes amongst which the pupil must search for the right one, (3) by informing him of classes which include the right one and which he would neglect if undirected, and (4) by calling his attention to the consequences of membership in this or that class. Thus (1) to ask a pupil 'What word does *arma* come from? What declension is it? What cases can it be?', makes the inference about *arma* easier than if he were left to an unsystematic trial of one translation after another. Thus (2) the question, 'What will prob-

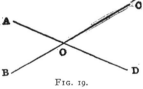

FIG. 19.

ably happen to Norfolk, Virginia, in the next thirty years?', is far too hard for eighth-grade pupils, but 'Which is the more likely, that Norfolk will increase its commerce or lose it?', is an appropriate question. Thus (3) the task of the pupil who is trying to prove as an original the proposition, 'If one straight line cuts another straight line the opposite angles are equal,' is made easier if he is told to think of all the angles of which angle AOB is a part and of all the angles of which angle COD is a part (see FIG. 19). (4) Help could have been given in the translation by suggesting that *arma* as accusative could find a place in the sentence as the object of *cano;* in the geometry original by pointing out that the angle BOC is equal to angle AOD; in the question about Norfolk by asking, 'What sort of a harbor has Norfolk? How near

164   *The Principles of Teaching*

is it to European ports? To the wheat fields of the west? To the coal and iron district of West Virginia?,' etc.

SUMMARY

Good inductive teaching selects representative particulars or instructive types for study, arranges them so that the pupil himself can realize their essential elements and derive the general truth, and requires its application to new particulars.

Good deductive teaching encourages the pupil to search for the proper class under which to put a fact, and directs his search by systematizing it, reducing alternatives and calling attention to neglected consequences.

In both cases good teaching uses comparison, contrast and analysis as the means of securing attention to the essential element and insists on the verification of conclusions by an appeal to known facts. In both cases a teacher's work is to fit the difficulty of the reasoning to the capacity of the pupil to think with parts and qualities.

The common error is to never teach reasoning but only the results of someone else's reasoning. When this is done after a make-believe process of reasoning which deceives the pupil into thinking he has himself solved the problem, the result is still worse.

§ 39. *Exercises*

1. Which of these interests is of assistance in teaching reasoning? The interest in the concrete, the interest in independent achievement, the interest in novelty.

2. Write a brief statement (from thirty to fifty words) of the influence of previous experience upon present reasoning.

Reasoning 165

3. What features of teaching that gain attention will be efficacious also in stimulating reasoning?

4. If the easiest way to satisfy teachers and succeed in school is by learning results rather than by understanding evidence, how much will students reason?

✓5. If in all his studies a student finds causes associated with their effects, conclusions with the evidence for them, facts with the elements which compose them, false inferences with denial, and the like, what will be the result by the general law of association?

6. Which two fundamental capacities are at the basis of reasoning? (See § 10.)

7. Should a teacher expect all high-school pupils to reason out the propositions in geometry or the translations in Latin ?

8. Show in a brief statement (of from fifty to a hundred words) that the principles of inductive teaching are simply adaptations of the principles of analysis.

9. Could a person reason well or follow intelligently a train of reasoning about a class of objects if his knowledge of the individual members of the class was imperfect?

10. Would he comprehend the answer to a question better if he were first made to realize the question? Why?

11. In which case would a student be the more likely to comprehend a theory or argument: if he had his knowledge in the form of images, for instance of a leaf of certain shape, or if he had it in the form of a judgment that the leaf was of that shape?

12. If all judgments refer eventually to real objects, will it be generally safe to trust that judgments can. be comprehended without actual demonstrations, experiments and object lessons?

13. When the right element or aspect of a fact is

166 *The Principles of Teaching*

selected, what more is necessary to secure the right conclusion?

14. Illustrate failures in reasoning in geometry, in grammar or in geography due to the absence of knowledge,—the absence, that is, of certain facts or connections between facts.

15. What devices would you use to make comparison easy in teaching the principle of the balance? In teaching the order of the sentence in German?

16. What are the differences between inductive reasoning and deductive reasoning? What are their resemblances?

17. Name a school subject which begins with and continues with general and abstract notions.

18. Name a school subject which deals almost exclusively with individual facts.

19. What grammar-school subject involves most deductive reasoning?

20. What high-school subject?

21. Recall the answers to the exercises on Analysis. Plan a lesson to teach inductively the law of falling bodies or the facts of electrolysis or the laws of the verb-forms in indirect discourse in Latin or the explanation of deltas.

22. Select ten sentences which would serve well as the individual facts from which to derive the general notions of active voice and passive voice.

23. Select ten which would be far less efficient.

24. How would you arrange the first ten on the blackboard for examination by the class?

25. Illustrate the use of contrast in teaching voice.

26. Arrange exercises suitable for the application of the knowledge gained of the active and passive voices.

Reasoning 167

27. Which will serve best as a type of a mammal, a cat or a whale? Why? A rabbit or a man? Why?

28. What experiment would you select as a typical illustration of the fact that heat is a mode of energy?

29. What are the defects of this lesson on tense?

"Tense is made to consist of six variations, viz., the present, the imperfect, the perfect, the pluperfect, and the first and second future tenses. The present tense represents an action or event, as passing at the time in which it is mentioned; as, "I rule; I am ruled." The imperfect tense represents an action or event, either as past and finished, or as remaining unfinished, at a certain time past; as, "I loved her; I was writing when he came." The perfect tense not only represents an event as past, but also conveys an allusion to the present tense; as, "I have finished my letter." The pluperfect tense represents a thing, not only as past, but as having past prior to some other point of time specified in the sentence; as, "I had finished writing before he arrived." The first future tense represents the action as yet to come, either with or without respect to the precise time; as, "I shall live; ye will see." The second future tense intimates that the action will be fully accomplished, at or before the time of another future action or event; as, "I shall have dined at one o'clock."

QUESTIONS.

How many variations of tense are there, and what are they? How does the present tense represent an action? How does the imperfect? How the perfect? How does the pluperfect? How does the first future? What is said of the second future?" [56]

30. In what ways is this better?

TENSES.

"345. Notice the following sets of sentences:—
    (1) Mr. Marshall *lives* in London.
        Mr. Marshall *lived* in York.
        Mr. Marshall *will live* in Naples.
    (2) Jack *is* in the playground now.

168   *The Principles of Teaching*

>   Jack *was* in school this morning.
>   Jack *will be* on the river this evening.

346.   Each verb gives us some notion of the time.

>   *Is* and *lives* speak of *present* time.
>   *Was* and *lived* speak of *past* time.
>   *Will be* and *will live* speak of *future* time.

347.   A Verb may thus have three times or TENSES— the Present, the Past, and the Future.

NOTE.—The term Present has already been used, as a name for certain of the Infinitives, Participles, and Gerunds (see page 145, footnote 1). As applied to Verbals, however, the term Present is inaccurate, as the time or tense belonging to a Present Infinitive, for example, depends upon the tense of the Verb in the sentence. Thus in the sentence, 'The last time you called you had to leave early,' the Present Infinitive *to leave* denotes an action now past, since it depends upon the Verb *had*, which is in the Past Tense. So with the Present Participle and the Present Gerund in these sentences: '*Going* down the street one day recently, I met old Mr. Crothers,' 'I was then in the habit of *walking* to my office.' In the same way, if a Present Verbal depends upon a Verb which is in the Future Tense, the Verbal becomes future in meaning; as, 'In case of my *finding* him at home, what shall I do?' 'If you will be there, *waiting* for him, he says he will not disappoint you,' 'We shall soon be ready *to start.*' " [57]

31.   In what ways is this better still?

Pick out the verbs in these sentences.

The boat now goes at eight o'clock, but next year it will make two trips, one at six and one at nine. This arrangement was made by the company at their last meeting. The residents had hoped for many months that better means of communication with the city would soon be established.

Why˙ do you call *goes, will make, was made, had hoped* and *would be established* verbs?

A verb may tell more than what somebody or something does or is. To-day we will find out one of the other things that a verb tells. Look at the verbs in the sen-

Reasoning 169

tences below and see what the difference is between those in the first column and those in the second.

The boat went yesterday.	The boat will go next year.
She sang that song Sunday.	She will sing it again to-morrow.
They were sick last week.	They will be sick for a few days longer.

Which of these verbs tell that something was in the past? Which verbs tell that something will be in the future?

Write two sentences about the action of a man going to New York. In the first tell about the man going to New York in the past; in the second tell about the man going to New York in the future.

Look at these sentences:

The train is going sixty miles an hour now.

Hear how loud that bird sings.

They are sick.

What other time is there besides the past and the future?

Tell in the case of each of these sentences whether the verb expresses a past action or a present action or a future action.

He will knock at your door at four o'clock.

He knocked at my door yesterday.

They write during this period.

He wrote a letter in the evening.

The wheels go around very fast.

They went around faster the other day.

What is the difference between the form of the verb 'knock' when it expresses or denotes future action and its form when it expresses or denotes past action? What is the difference between the form of the verb write when it denotes present action and its form when it denotes past action? What word is used to tell about a person going in the past? To tell about a person going now?

Verbs tell not only the kind of action or event but also the time when it takes place. The form of the verb is different when the action or event is represented in the past from what it is when the action or event is represented in the present or in the future.

170 *The Principles of Teaching*

A difference in the form of a verb to denote time is called Tense.

A verb that denotes present action is in the Present Tense.

A verb that denotes past action is in the Past Tense.

A verb that denotes future action is in the Future Tense.

Write under each verb in the sentences below what tense it is in (as is done in the first line).

It is hotter this summer than it was last summer. It will
present   past
be cold enough in the winter. The sun will rise later and set earlier. Evening came so soon last November that the lights were being lit in the house when I reached home from school. We do not light them now till after seven. You can see that it is quite light now though the bells are ringing seven.

Did they send up my trunk from the station? No. They would not promise that it should be sent without a check. If you will send them the check, it will be sent. I shall be passing the office this evening, anyway. Won't it be open? It used to be open evenings.

Write two sentences each with a verb in the present tense.

Write two sentences each with a verb in the past tense.

Write two sentences each with a verb in the future tense.

32. What advantage would a student gain by making for himself the figure and statement given below (FIG. 20 A) as a means toward doing this problem? A lady is buying carpet to carpet a room 14 feet long and 11 feet wide. She has already a border of carpet one foot wide all around the room. How many square yards of carpet must she buy?

33. What are the essential elements in the student's knowledge about the inside rectangle which enable him to find how many square yards it contains?

34. What properties or consequences or associates of

108 square feet or of 9 feet long and 12 feet long must be called up in his mind to carry him on toward the solution?

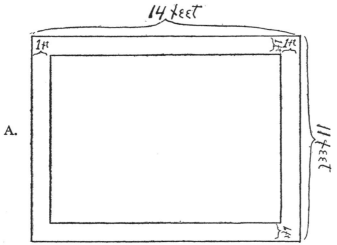

A.

How many square yards is the inner rectangle?

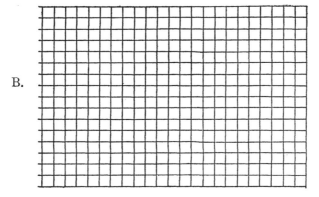

B.

FIG. 20.

172   *The Principles of Teaching*

35. How would the lady have verified the correctness of her decision? How might the pupil do so conveniently with a piece of squared paper like FIG. 20 B?

36. How would students in geometry get on with the proposition, 'Lines parallel to the same straight line are parallel to each other,' if it were stated as, 'Two lines are parallel to the same straight line: what of it?' Why?

37. How would they succeed with it if they thought of the two lines only as straight lines, as each making an

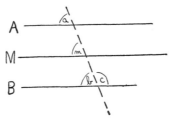

FIG. 21.

PROOF. Suppose T a transversal, making corresponding angles a, m, b, with A, M, B, respectively.
Since A is parallel to M, angle a = angle m. A line cutting two parallels makes corresponding angles equal.
And since B is parallel to M, angle b = angle m.
Therefore angle a = angle b.
Therefore A is parallel to B. If two corresponding angles are equal, the nes are parallel.

angle equal to two right angles, as not meeting each other or the third straight line? Why?

38. How would they succeed if they thought of the three lines as cut by a transversal, but did not think of the relationships of equality and supplementalness of the angles made where parallels are cut by a transversal? Why?

39. Under what class should they think of angle a?

40. Under what class should they think of angle b?

41. What property of things equal to the same thing furthers the demonstration?

Reasoning 173

42. Classify the following helps in the case of the proposition just described as:

    1. Systematizing the search.

    2. Reducing alternatives.

    3. Suggesting a useful alternative.

    4. Suggesting consequences.

a. After drawing lines A and B parallel to line M, draw a transversal cutting all three.

b. Examine the relations of the angles thus formed.

c. Which is the more likely to help you, to prove angle (a) equal to angle (b) or to prove angle (a) supplementary to angle (c)?

d. If you could prove that angle (a) equalled angle (b) could you then prove line A parallel to line B?

43. Make a list of suggestions or questions designed to guide a 7th or 8th grade pupil in solving problem A. (The most instructive way to do so will be to actually assign the problem to some pupil and then help him to conquer those difficulties which he actually experiences in trying to solve it, making notes of the forms your help takes.)

44. State in the case of each of your suggestions and questions how and why it was of help.

A.

John left Central Square at 9 A. M., riding a bicycle whose wheels were each 30 inches in diameter, and rode for two hours, pedalling at such a rate as to make ninety revolutions of the rear wheel per minute. After stopping 20 minutes to rest he continued, but at a rate only two-thirds as fast. Fred started from Central Square at 10 A. M., followed the same route as A for one hour, then rode a mile off the road and a mile back again. He then continued after John. His wheel was so geared that each revolution of the crank shaft carried him the same

174 *The Principles of Teaching*

distance as a wheel of 72 inches diameter would carry anyone in a single revolution. He pedalled throughout at such a rate as to make 36 revolutions of the crank shaft per minute. How far behind John would he be at 12 o'clock?

45. Give two suggestions or questions designed to reduce alternatives in the search for the classes under which to think of coal, heat, steam, pressure, and so on, so as to demonstrate why a few tons of coal can move a heavy train for miles.

46. Illustrate the use of comparison or contrast in directing attention to the essential element in the case of the fact, *heated water,* namely, its force of expansion.

47. Criticise (A) and (B) on the basis of the facts of this chapter and the preceding one.

48. Suggest modifications of (A) and of (B) with a view to adding clearness, omitting irrelevant facts, bringing the essentials into relief, and applying the general truth taught.

A.

"44. ATTRACTION OF GRAVITATION.—As the attraction of cohesion unites the particles of matter into masses or bodies, so the attraction of gravitation tends to force these masses towards each other, to form those of still greater dimensions. The term gravitation, does not here strictly refer to the weight of bodies, but to the attraction of the masses of matter towards each other, whether downwards, upwards, or horizontally.

45. The attraction of gravitation is mutual, since all bodies not only attract other bodies, but are themselves attracted.

46. Two cannon balls, when suspended by long cords, so as to hang quite near each other, are found to exert a mutual attraction, so that neither of the cords is ex-

A.

actly perpendicular, but they approach each other as in Fig. A.

47. In the same manner, the heavenly bodies, when they approach each other, are drawn out of the line of their paths, or orbits, by mutual attraction.

48. The force of attraction increases in proportion as bodies approach each other, and by the same law it must diminish in proportion as they recede from each other.

49. Attraction, in technical language, is inversely as the squares of the distances between the two bodies. That is, in proportion as the square of the distance increases, in the same proportion attraction decreases, and so the contrary. Thus, if at the distance of 2 feet, the attraction be equal to 4 pounds, at the distance of 4 feet, it will be only 1 pound; for the square of 2 is 4, and the square of 4 is 16, which is four times the square of 2. On the contrary, if the attraction at the distance of 6 feet be 3 pounds, at the distance of 2 feet it will be 9 times as much, or 27 pounds, because 36, the square of 6, is equal to 9 times 4, the square of 2.

50. The intensity of light is found to increase and diminish in the same proportion. Thus, if a board a foot square, be placed at the distance of one foot from a candle, it will be found to hide the light from another board of two feet square, at the distance of two feet from the candle. Now a board of two feet square is just four times as large as one of one foot square, and therefore the light at double the distance being spread over 4 times the surface, has only one-fourth the intensity.

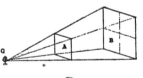

B.

51. The experiment may be easily tried, or may be readily understood by Fig. B. where c represents the candle, A, the small board, and B the large one; B being four times the size of A.

The force of the attraction of gravitation is in proportion to the quantity of matter the attracting body contains.

176   *The Principles of Teaching*

Some bodies of the same bulk contain a much greater quantity of matter than others; thus, a piece of lead contains about twelve times as much matter as a piece of cork of the same dimensions, and therefore a piece of lead of any given size, and a piece of cork twelve times as large, will attract each other equally." [58]

B.

"15. THE LAW OF GRAVITATION.—We all know these facts: that all bodies near the earth fall to it if they are free to fall; that all bodies on the earth are held on it by some means which we cannot see; and that the earth, the moon, and the planets are all held in place and kept moving about the sun, also by some invisible means. We see at a glance that there must be some mighty power, some great force necessary to accomplish this. And we call this the force of *gravitation.*

But scientific men have gone a step farther; and they tell us that *all* bodies of matter exert this same force,— *that every body of matter in the universe attracts every other body with a certain amount of force.* The strength of this attraction between two bodies increases with the amount of matter in them, and decreases as they are moved farther apart.

The rate of increase and decrease has been measured in many cases, and the result is summed up in the so-called *Law of Gravitation.* The law is as follows:

The strength of the attraction of gravitation between any two bodies of matter varies directly with the product of their masses (quantity of matter), and inversely as the squares of the distance between their centers of attraction.

Or, putting it a little more simply, when a body attracts two others, for example, the greater of the two will be drawn by a force as much larger than the other as its mass is times the mass of the lesser. The last part of the law means that as the square of the distance between two bodies increases, for instance, the attraction between them decreases in proportion. In computing the relative

Reasoning 177

attraction of two bodies for a third, of course both *distance* and *quantity of matter* must be considered. Thus we find, for example, that while the mass of the sun is far greater than that of the moon, still the moon's distance is so much less than the sun's that it attracts bodies at the earth's surface more strongly than the sun does. This is shown by the tides, which are governed rather more by the moon's position than by the sun's.

16 Gravity.—We wonder, almost at once, why, if every body of matter attracts every other, all things are not drawn together in one place. The reason is simple. If the strength of attraction increases with the amount of matter, surely the attraction of *the earth* is stronger than that of any body on its surface. Even if two bodies rest on a perfectly level surface, the attraction for the earth will still be so great that they cannot come together; for in moving towards each other they will rub on the surface hard enough to overcome the weak attraction between them.

The experiment has been made of hanging two heavy iron balls near together from a great height; it was found that they moved towards each other a very little (Fig. a). In so doing, however, it is clear that the balls must swing up just a little from their lowest position; in other words, the attractive force of each for the other must be great enough to raise them a little way against the force of gravity. For this reason only very heavy masses will so swing toward each other, and even they will not move far from the vertical line.

Now we see why bodies fall: it is because they are *pulled* down by a force. And this force is only one of the 'properties' which all matter has in common. The earth, being so much larger and so near, exerts this force more strongly than any other body, so that all things on the earth stay on it or fall toward it when free to fall. When we are speaking of this attraction with reference to the earth, we call it gravity. If it were not for this force of gravity, no moving body would remain long on

12

178 *The Principles of Teaching*

the earth. We should jump up and keep on going, toss up our hats and never see them again. A ball would stay as well beneath a shelf as on top of it; in fact, we should have no need of shelves, for things would stay anywhere." [59]

For Further Reading

C. A. McMurry and F. M. McMurry, *The Method of the Recitation,* Chapters VII-XIV inclusive.

W. James, *Talks to Teachers on Psychology,* Chapter XIII.

CHAPTER XI

RESPONSES OF CONDUCT: MORAL TRAINING

Preparatory, *Elements of Psychology,* §§ 50-55

§ 40. *Education and Conduct*

The springs of conduct are the instincts given by nature and the ideas given by education. The actual direction which the stream of behavior takes is represented by the habits one acquires. "The good and efficient character implies the subjugation of those instinctive tendencies to action which injure oneself or others, the energetic action of desirable ones, the presence of worthy ideals and the connection of these with appropriate acts, a multiplicity of useful habits, the power to see and react to the element of a situation which will issue in an act producing the best results, the power to react to barren abstractions such as *ought, right* and *true,* the power to delay decision until enough evidence is in to warrant one in deciding, the power to refrain from delaying it too long, and the power to stand the strain of effort implied in choosing a relatively unattractive course of behavior.

"**The Elements of Moral Training.**—The training of character is correspondingly complex. Useful instincts must be given a chance to exercise themselves and become habits. Harmful instinctive responses must be inhibited through lack of stimulus, through the substitution of desirable ones or through actual resultant discomfort, as

180   The Principles of Teaching

best fits each special case. The mind must be supplied
with noble ideas through the right examples at home, in
school, in the world at large and in books. These ideas
must be made to issue in appropriate action or they may
be worse than useless. The capacity to examine any
situation and see what the essential fact in it which should
decide action is, must be constantly exercised and guided.
The habits of letting 'It is right' or 'It is best' or 'It will
be for the real welfare of the world' or the like, be an
absolutely final warrant for action must be firmly fixed.
The will must be prevented alike from precipitate responses and from dawdling indecision. The power to
banish from mind attractive but unworthy ideas, and to
go on one's way regardless of the effort involved in so
doing, must be gradually built up. Especially important
is the actual formation of definite habits. If a man does
what is useful and right he will soon gain proper ideas
of social efficiency and of morals. If he learns to do the
right thing in a thousand particular situations, he will, so
far as he has the capacity, gain the power to see what act
a new situation demands. If he is made to obey a thousand particular 'This is right's' and 'That is right's' he
will, so far as he has the capacity, come to connect
respect and obedience with the abstractly right and true.
If he does what he has to do well and treats his fellow
beings as he should in the thousands of situations of the
ordinary course of life, he will gain the power to conquer attractive counter-impulses." [60]

Moral Training in Schools.—The problem of moral
training in day schools is still further complicated by the
fact that pupils are under the teacher's control only one-
fourth of their waking hours, that there are thirty or
forty different moral natures for one teacher to help, that

Responses of Conduct: Moral Training 181

the present demands of schools in the shape of intellectual education reduce moral training to an incident, a by-product, of school work. A teacher is also limited in the means at his disposal for moral training. The tone of the family, the treatment received from friends, public opinion and practice, and hopes and fears of supernatural intervention in life or after death have been and are the chief means of moral influence. Of the four, the teacher can count only upon the second to the extent that he himself wins the position of a friend and upon the third to the extent that he can by the selection of pupils, by wise legislation and by personal influence modify the tone of the school or class. Finally, many of the desirable traits of character can get exercise only in the duties and temptations of real life. The special morality of employer and employee, of buyer and seller, of husband and wife, of parents and children or of ruler and ruled requires in each case more than a school-room full of children as its adequate stimulus.

The answer to the question, 'How can a teacher make his pupils all good and efficient?,' is, 'He cannot.' To expect school education to determine moral development is like expecting a city water-supply to abolish all sickness. The one is a psychological impossibility as truly as the other is a physical impossibility. The real problem for the teacher in the day schools is rather, 'How can I, without neglect of the demands for intellectual training made by the government or parents that employ me, do a little of what so much needs to be done for the moral training of these boys and girls?' The teacher, that is, needs to study the principles of teaching with respect to moral character under the limitations of school life, since in the case of moral training these limiting conditions are

182   *The Principles of Teaching*

of as much practical importance as the general principles.

The Fundamental Laws of Teaching in the Sphere of Conduct.—The general principles come from the law of instinct, the law of habit formation, the law of selective thinking and the law of suggestion.

The application of the laws of instinct and of habit formation to connections of conduct was clearly made in Chapters III, IV, V and VIII. Suffice it to note here that it is even more desirable in the moral than in the intellectual life to substitute an opposite good or harmless tendency for a bad instinctive response, rather than to rely solely on punishment; and that it is even riskier in the moral life than in the intellectual to expect that a situation will produce its right response unless that response has been put with the situation in actual conduct and rewarded with satisfaction.

The law of selective thinking applied to conduct is: What you will do in the face of any given fact depends upon what element or aspect of that fact you select. The union laborer who throws a stone at the strike-breaker if he thinks of the element, 'scab worker who cuts my wages' may stop and argue with him if he thinks of the element 'one of the enemy's forces, who may be won over to our side.' The schoolboys celebrating an athletic victory respond to the proposal to tear down Jones' fence by tearing it down if they think only of the aspect, 'celebrate by a bonfire'; by passing it by if they think only of the aspect, 'destroying the property of a poor old workman who often comes out to see us practice.'

The same situation may cause different acts according to what element of it the law of partial activity selects; hence one means of securing right acts is to teach children to think of that element in a situation which is morally the essential one. To think of copying another's

Responses of Conduct: Moral Training 183

work as 'stealing' may make the habit impossible to many pupils who practiced it without hesitation so long as they thought of it as 'what everyone does.' Hence to reveal the true moral meaning of copying may be enough to prevent it. The occasional faults and failures of children who are in general well disposed are very often failures to select the morally essential element, to put the situation in the proper class, to call it by its right name.

From the law of suggestion, that 'any idea tends to result in its appropriate act if no competing idea or physical impediment prevents,' is derived the principle that in so far as the important thing is to get the right act done and in so far as the comprehension of why it is right and the decision to perform it are relatively unimportant, to that extent suggestion is an efficient means of moral influence. To distract the mind of a six year old from the ideas that make him cowardly,—to encourage him to be brave by telling him that he *is* brave,—may thus be a better moral training than arguments about the folly of fear, which he cannot appreciate, or a rebuke for his cowardice, which only gives him the idea of being so. To take it for granted that high-school students expect to be honorable,—to arouse the virtues of the gentleman and of the lady by behaving as if they already existed,— is likely to be better teaching than any form of argument or legislation.

This same principle implies the folly of any extended discussion of wrong acts which would be done only rarely and by a few members of a class. Such a discussion is more likely to suggest the act to pupils who would otherwise never have committed it than to prevent it in those who otherwise would. The parent's 'Do not ever put the fish-hooks in your ears,' and the teacher's, 'I hope

184 *The Principles of Teaching*

that no boy in my school will ever cut a live dog open to see its liver,' will thus do more harm than good!

Limitations Due to School Conditions.—The limitations which the conditions of school life set to the application of these principles should be obvious. The first are those due to numbers. John needs opportunities for the display of courage, but two-thirds of the class need to reduce their rashness. The majority must be taught to think of other pupils as possessors of rights, but cringing, weak Jennie needs to think of the element, 'no better than I.' Half need the suggestion of sympathy and good fellowship, but a few mean and cruel ones need stern justice and the surety that you, their teacher, know them to be bullies and will see that they get the treatment which bullies deserve.

There are also those due to lack of complete control. The life of the home and street gives or withholds the stimuli to many of the instincts, good and bad, forms almost exclusively the habits of behavior toward money, sex and many other important aspects of life, and also the habits of selection of elements to be acted on in the majority of moral situations. It also furnishes incessantly moral or immoral suggestions through those most powerful of all suggestive forces, the example and works of human beings.

The third limitation is due to the fact that the intellectual changes which teachers are expected to make in pupils demand nearly all of the time at the school's disposal. If five hours of Monday could be spent in such works of unselfishness as collecting flowers for a hospital, if Tuesdays could be spent in the care of younger children, if on Wednesdays each pupil could be led to work and play under the guidance of honor and justice, and so on through the week, an efficient teacher could

Responses of Conduct: Moral Training 185

form the characters of her class as she can now form their intellects. But learning lessons and doing experiments are at best inconvenient ways of forming the moral habits needed in life and at the worst are of no direct moral value at all.

That the opportunities of the teacher for moral training are fewer than he might wish is no excuse for their neglect. On the contrary efficient teaching will be the more careful to utilize those which do exist and not to waste any precious time or energy by depending on faulty principles.

The opportunities of the school may be grouped as: (1) opportunities for training in moral action itself through behavior in the class-room and in connection with other school activities over which the teacher has some degree of control, (2) opportunities for specific moral instruction other than training in moral action itself, and (3) opportunities for training in moral appreciation and ideals through the regular school studies.

§ 41. *School Habits as Moral Training*

The Range of School Morality.—Although the school is not the main cause of children's conduct and is limited in its action on the moral life in many ways, it still can influence somewhat almost every moral habit. Athletic competitions may be a school of honor and justice; the school recess may be a training class in the social virtues of courtesy, sympathy and good fellowship; habits of cleanliness of body and dress may be acquired in every school day. School banks for thrift, street-cleaning clubs for civic patriotism, school newspapers for teaching proper control of public expressions of opinion, and school contributions to charities, are samples of the many

186 *The Principles of Teaching*

ways in which efficient teachers use school life for training in moral conduct.

Discipline in the Narrow Sense.— The moral habits connected with school work in the narrower sense,—the results of school discipline,—though of narrow range, are given constant practice and, like the equally narrow training of office, factory, army life or professional duties, may contribute important elements of character. The habits of punctuality, work, thoroughness, submission of one's own impulses to the general good, of expecting a just reward for one's deeds, acting for the future as well as the present and fitting behavior to reality rather than to foolish fears and hopes—such results of wise school discipline have a real moral value.

To obtain this value, however, the aim of school discipline must be made the moral welfare of the pupils rather than the convenience of the teacher. Offenses against other pupils must be considered as objectionable as offenses against the teacher. The success of discipline must be measured by the sum of positive well doing more than by the absence of bad behavior. The virtues of boyhood and girlhood must not be made subservient to the virtues of the class-room. Obedience and zeal in school duties must not be put on a pinnacle above honor, kindness, justice and courage.

To the general principles of § 40 one further principle for school discipline may be added. Avoid making rules involving distinctions which the pupils cannot make. 'No communication between pupils without special permission except in the five minutes recesses between periods,' a ten-year-old can understand; the distinction between a period and the five minutes recess is easy. But 'No communication between pupils that disturbs the work of the class' will be beyond him. Mr. A. C. Benson

Responses of Conduct: Moral Training 187

relates that a boy who was rebuked for putting a dormouse down the neck of of a very easy-going master, asked in all good faith, 'But how was I to know that he drew the line at a dormouse?' Rules which vary in complex ways with attendant circumstances or with the motive for the act are unsuitable for young children and for the duller older children. Moral as well as intellectual progress should be made step by step along clear pathways.

§ 42. Specific Moral Instruction

Moral Stimulation a Means, Not an End.—Morality consists of habits of action and there is no sure way to secure habits of action but by action. We become truthful by telling the truth, courageous by facing the danger. The cure for stinginess is to give; for cruelty, acts of mercy and kindness. Ideas of the right and desires to do the right are valuable only as steps toward actually doing it. To learn what is right and reject it removes one a step further from virtue than he was before. To desire to do a certain worthy act and yet come no nearer doing it is to form one of the most immoral of habits, that of wasting one's moral emotions. Specific moral instruction, whether it be a calm scientific discussion of what is good and of what consequently our duty is, or a passionate inspiration to better ideals through the appreciation of concrete cases of heroism, self-denial, honor and love, is only a means toward the end, moral action.

The Value of Specific Instruction.—How useful a means such specific instruction as may be given in schools is, nobody knows. It is universal in French schools, and very rare in this country; yet no one has traced to school training any moral superiority of French over American

188   *The Principles of Teaching*

life. It is heartily advocated by many thoughtful people and laughed at by others equally thoughtful.

To some extent it is true, as the latter would claim, that one's moral life, like one's digestion, gets on best when one thinks as little as possible about it. Just as to go outdoors, to take exercise and to eat plain food are good for the digestion but to think about what to do for it is extremely bad, so, they would say, to do what you ought is good for your moral life, but to think about what is good for it, is bad for it. Moreover acute students of human nature are more and more leaning toward the doctrine that conduct influences our feelings more than feelings influence conduct. 'Act toward your neighbor as you would toward yourself and you will come to love him' is as true as, 'Love your neighbor as yourself and you will come to act rightly toward him,' they tell us. For a boy to learn to appreciate honor and as a consequence to tell the truth is, they would say, not so common a sequence as for a boy to tell the truth and as a consequence to learn to appreciate honor. Some would go so far as to assert that the only moral sentiments worth having were sentiments which came as a result of right action. 'A man's conscience is not the producer but the product of his career.'

On the other hand it may safely be said that (1) on the basis of their natural moral tendencies and previous moral experiences children can be taught what is right for the same reasons that they can be taught what is true; that (2) interests can be aroused in being honorable and just and kind for the same reasons that interests can be aroused in being well-informed and skillful; and that (3) while nothing save conduct can finally determine character, the ideas and insight which specific school instruction

Responses of Conduct: Moral Training 189

in morality can give may be most useful stimuli to right conduct.

§ 43. *The Moral Effects of School Studies*

The advocates of each school subject are fond of asserting that it not only gives valuable knowledge and habits of thought but also strengthens the will and enlightens the conscience. If we are to believe them arithmetic makes you truthful; science makes you patient; geography makes you love your neighbors in the Philippines as yourself; history makes you humble and brave and honorable; literature stirs every noble emotion and gives birth to all the virtues.

There is no doubt that the primarily intellectual work of learning the school subjects does produce secondarily certain moral results. But there is also no doubt that such statements as those given are gross exaggerations. It is necessary in estimating the moral effect of any study to bear in mind: (1) That a certain habit formed in connection with a school subject will rarely extend far beyond it. We must not base hopes of moral education upon the false dogma of formal discipline (see Chapter XV). (2) That there is a fundamental difference between getting ideas of what is good and wishing to be good. The first is a response of knowledge; the second, of attitude. (3) That there is an equal difference between wishing to be good and being good. The latter is a response not of attitude, but of action. (4) That the aesthetic emotions do not necessarily or even often predispose to their real counterparts. A boy may read tales of courage with appreciation and still be timid; a girl

190 *The Principles of Teaching*

may adore a virtue in the heroine and practice its opposite none the less the next day.

With these four warnings to preserve us from over-estimating the moral effect of studies and from expecting it in the wrong places, a just idea may be obtained of what the school studies can do for moral education and of how they may be taught so as to fulfill that function.

The Semi-Moral Habits.—Intellectual-moral habits such as accuracy, thoughtfulness, persistence, patience, neglect of necessary discomfort and intellectual justice or open-mindedness, can be cultivated through school work. These habits are primarily restricted to the special data with which they are acquired and the extent to which they evolve into general habits will depend upon the principles stated later in the chapter on Formal Discipline. The principles for teaching with respect to them are the same as for purely intellectual habits and have been sufficiently treated in Chapters III, IV, V and VIII. No one study should have a monopoly of these semi-intellectual virtues. It may be most convenient to teach accuracy in arithmetic but it should be taught in every lesson about facts. Perhaps one can learn history without securing a gain in open-mindedness such as physical science gives, but he ought not to.

Geography.—Knowledge of the life of man such as is given in geography and general reading, though it by no means implies sympathy and justice toward one's fellows or efforts to be like the best, does have moral value, because a certain amount of wrong-doing is due not to ill-will but to ignorance. The mistaken philanthropy which sends flannel night-gowns to equatorial negroes, the careless folly which insults the deepest feelings of the Chinese by removing ancestral tombs to make way for a railway, the narrow-minded prudery which insists on European habits of dress and conduct in the South Sea

Responses of Conduct: Moral Training 191

islanders and thereby destroys a natural and true modesty—these are all faults which knowledge should have cured. Moreover, one cure for the vices of suspicion, irrational hatred and careless neglect and one means to the virtues of social spirit, cooperation and sympathy is mutual acquaintance. For the rich to know the life of the poor, for the employer to know the life of his employees, for the American to know the life of the German, for the European to know the life of the Asiatic—is a moral as well as an intellectual gain.

History and Literature.—The study of human life in biographies and history serves morality by teaching two great lessons: the first, that on the whole and in the long run public esteem is given to moral greatness, not to wealth or position or success; the second, that the world is more than a place where you eat and sleep and endure work for the sake of a few cheap animal pleasures, that it is full of great issues, unselfish motives and heroic deeds. It also presents moral incentives in the efficient form of attractive ideals of character and action.

To realize that to the great judge, the future, and to the best people of the present, character far outweighs material success or social prestige is possible for even a ten-year-old child and may be a real source of conduct for boys and girls in their 'teens. It reinforces the wisdom of the better homes and offsets the vulgar emphasis of material success in the worse. To learn concretely day by day that the rich of the past are not worthy of mention, that the powerful are judged by the ways they gained and used their power, that what men do for others is the measure of true success—this may mean for many boys and girls a changed moral judgment, a new insight into the moral essentials of their own conduct.

192 *The Principles of Teaching*

The life of the average household and of the average community is necessarily commonplace. It may be morally good or it may be sordid and bestial, but it is in either case commonplace. It does not enlarge the range of effort or stir the mind; it excites to only the conventional virtues or vices. The conventionally good and the conventionally bad alike need to learn of the great moral problems that men and women have had to face and of the acts of faith and love and honor and duty and courage and sacrifice which have enriched the world. For those who have known only the commonplace good, the good needs to be made a great and important and inspiring fact. For those who have known chiefly the sordid and vulgar side of life, history and biographies supply a new faith in life and hope for the future.

A word of warning is necessary here. To give something beyond the commonplace must not be to demean the commonplace. The honest day's work of the laborer, the cleanliness and thrift of the housewife, mere honesty with respect to money, avoidance of quarreling, speaking well of one's neighbors, supporting the church and the other common duties of the common man's life are as valuable morally as the martyr's choice of death, the hero's renunciation of wealth and fame or the stand of the three hundred at Marathon. If learning the goodness of the great were to weaken respect for the steady virtues of the many, it had better remain unknown. Indeed to show the real dignity of the ordinary moral acts, their essential community with the rare and exciting heroisms of history, and to enforce the lesson that the character acquired by everyday conduct is the character that conquers in great emergencies and crises, is an essential element of good teaching of the moral aspect of history.

Responses of Conduct: Moral Training 193

For all of us the most efficient presentation of a moral principle is usually through a personal life, and for children that is almost the only way. They live morally by models far more than by rules. The boy can try to be like Washington and Lincoln and Lee who could hardly understand and would soon forget a description of patriotism. It is then no small advantage that history can fill the mind with noble ideals, and make it acquainted with characters in whose presence the flippant excuses and tawdry ambitions of weak men and women seem unworthy of attention.

The study of human life in literature has in general the same moral influence as in history and biography. The differences are that the moral lessons from literature are less vigorous (especially to older students) in so far as they are felt as matters of fiction, but are simpler and hence clearer, and are of wider range.

The best methods of securing the moral values of geography, history and literature are not surely known. Our grandparents were taught to make solemn reflections on their duties; our parents had the moral of each event clearly pointed out; the best present practice is to allow or encourage such comments by the pupils as are expressions of real feeling but never to force them. There is something to be said in favor of leaving the subject matter of literature to speak for itself and permitting moral deductions only from facts. It is risky to teach children, 'Thinking too much of revenge is bad; see what happened to Shylock,' for the feeling of the unreality of the fiction which will sooner or later come will tend to diffuse over the maxim itself. Moreover it is a bad habit to use anything but facts as a reason for anything. The risk is not, however, so great as it seems logically to be, for with little children

194 *The Principles of Teaching*

the maxim may be kept and the illogical reason for it forgotten, and with anyone who can distinguish fact from fiction the illogical reason is usually thought of only as a suggestion or illustration, not as a reason at all. The high-school girl does not think, 'Revenge is bad because Shylock found it to be so,' but more nearly, 'Revenge is bad for reasons with which I am not now concerned; the tale of Shylock is a striking illustration in fiction.'

In closing this chapter I venture to remind the reader that, quite apart from moral influences through direct training in conduct, specific lessons about morality and the moral significance of the usual school studies, school education has a high moral value. To give anyone some useful work to do in the world is in itself to help him morally. The school is thus a moral force by securing useful intellectual activity and encouraging habits of efficient work and worthy interests for leisure hours. Even though a school should restrict its direct aim to intellectual training and should never say a word or do a thing about virtues and vices, it would still make for morality in the sense that labor in business or in the household or impersonal activities of any sort make for morality.

§ 44. *Exercises*

1. What are some instincts which have a moral as well as or instead of an intellectual significance?

2. Write, in from seventy-five to one hundred and twenty-five words, a statement of the principles of habit formation as applied to moral education.

3. Recall your answers to Exercises 39, 40 and 41, of § 29.

4. Give two illustrations of wrong acts due to responding to the wrong element or aspect of a situation.

Responses of Conduct: Moral Training 195

5. How may the law of selective thinking explain the common fact of two people, both of the highest morality, acting in opposite ways with respect to a certain moral issue?

6. How may the same fact be explained by the fact of apperception, *i. e.*, the fact of differences in knowledge in the two individuals?

7. What criticism would you make of discussing the impropriety of suicide in a text-book on morality for boys and girls? This is done in some French text-books.

8. What principle of psychological fact supports the following recommendations made in Fitch's *Lectures on Teaching?*

'To say "I ought to be obeyed" is to invite him to discuss the grounds of your authority, perhaps to dispute it.' [61]

'It is not well in laying down a school rule to say anything about the penalty which will fall upon those who transgress it.' [62]

9. Do you think it would be well to have, as the French schools do, regular text-books on morality? Write from thirty to sixty words justifying your answer.

10. What will be the probable moral effect on pupils of each of these practices?

a. Punishing an entire class for the offense of one or a few.

b. So-called 'putting children on their honor,' *i. e.*, requiring that they themselves at the close of the day or week tell whether or not they have broken school rules.

c. Making the general docility and good behavior of a child a partial determinant of the mark given him for scholarship.

11. Into what two groups would you divide the following acts of a girl in school?

196 *The Principles of Teaching*

    a. Whispering without permission.
    b. Tormenting a younger child.
    c. Stealing candy.
    d. Eating it in school.
    e. Tardiness.
    f. Cheating.
    g. Laziness.

12. What is the essential difference between the two groups?

13. What difference should be made in the treatment of the two groups besides greater severity for the more serious offenses?

14. A number of parents, teachers and children were asked the question, 'What is the worst fault in children?' The parents said most often, 'Disobedience'; the children, 'Cruelty'; and the teachers 'Lying and Inattention.' What is the relaton between 'troublesome to me' and 'wrong' in the mind of the average person?

15. Should the rewards and punishments of school be administered for the sake of the convenience of the teacher or for the sake of the moral development of the scholar?

16. Give one or two illustrations of violations of the principle implied in your answer?

17. What moral loss is supposed to come from permitting students to help each other in their work?

18. What moral gain might come from permitting and even encouraging mutual aid?

19. Why are the activities of the recess period, of the athletic field and of student organizations especially important for moral training?

20. Name four or five ways in which real moral action outside of class-room duties can be stimulated and directed by the school without making impracticable demands upon the time and energy of teachers.

Responses of Conduct: Moral Training   197

21. What paragraph in § 40 states the same doctrine as the last sentence of this quotation:

"How is it when an alternative is presented to you for choice, and you are uncertain what you ought to do? You first hesitate, and then·you deliberate. And in what does your deliberation consist? It consists in trying to apperceive the case successively by a number of different ideas, which seem to fit it more or less, until at last you hit on one which seems to fit it exactly. If that be an idea which is a customary forerunner of action in you, which enters into one of your maxims of positive be· havior, your hesitation ceases, and you act immediately. If, on the other hand, it be an idea which carries inaction as its habitual result, if it ally itself with *prohibition,* then you unhesitatingly refrain. The problem is, you see, to find the right idea or conception for the case." [63]

Professor James says in one of his lectures:

"This leads to a fourth maxim. Don't preach too much to your pupils or abound in good talk in the abstract. Lie in wait rather for the practical opportunities, be prompt to seize those as they pass, and thus at one operation get your pupils both to think, to feel and to do. The strokes of *behavior* are what give the new set to the character, and work the good habits into its organic tissue. Preaching and talking too soon become an ineffectual bore." [64]

22. How much preaching is 'too much'?

23. What are some of the 'practical opportunities' of the school for moral training?

24. Why is it 'the strokes of *behavior*' that give the new set to the character?

For Further Reading

E. A. Kirkpatrick, *Fundamentals of Child Study,* Chapter XI.

W. James, *Talks to Teachers on Psychology,* Chapter XV, and pp. 229-301.

H. Spencer, *Education,* Chapter III.

J. MacCunn, *The Making of Character.*

CHAPTER XII

Responses of Feeling

§ 45. *The Real Emotions*

The general laws which control responses of thought and of action control also responses of feeling. The work of education is to preserve desirable instinctive emotional responses by giving them exercise and rewarding them with pleasure, to eliminate the unfit ones and to form habits of feeling the right feeling at the right time. The principles stated in the chapters on instinct, interest, apperception and habit are then applicable to the emotions. Since their application will be clear from previous chapters, the present chapter will state only the special principles peculiar to responses of feeling.

Instincts of Emotional Response.—Some of the most beneficent qualities of human nature are given by nature in the instincts of sympathy, affection, courage, joy and maternal love. Social life is based largely on these. They are too precious to be lost by disuse or by careless education. Although life outside the school must always be chiefly responsible for the cultivation of these virtues, the school should make the most of what opportunities it does have. If the life of the class-room is destitute of sympathy, happiness, courage and love, it is offering a pitifully incomplete education. Good teaching will provide exercise for these instinctive emotions as well as for the native intellectual capacities.

Responses of Feeling

So also envy, jealousy, fear, delight in cruelty and the like must be eliminated as well as ignorance or disobedience. Good teaching will substitute honest rivalry and sympathy for envy and jealousy and inhibit delight in cruelty by cultivating the opposing habits of care and protection.

Ambition, pride, anger and the other emotions which are good or bad according to their objects should be directed as carefully as the capacities to observe, remember and argue. To hate aright is as necessary as to infer aright. "The great secret of education," says Adam Smith, "is to direct vanity to proper objects." [65]

Habits of Emotional Response.—To arouse a given emotion in connection with a given situation, *e. g.*, to make a person feel gratitude at the thought of the revolutionary heroes, we may use one of three methods. (1) Ideas that have in the past been connected with the emotion may be aroused. For instance a teacher properly expects an announcement of a favorite excursion to be greeted with joy. (2) The emotion may be communicated through imitation. If the teacher and half of the class are thrilled with admiration for a member of the class who has honorably confessed his unfairness toward a classmate, the rest of the class will be more likely to admire him also. (3) The bodily response characteristic of the emotion may be aroused. Let the frightened one walk steadily toward the enemy, looking him square in the eye, shouting in a loud voice, "I'm not afraid of you, I'll eat you alive," and brandishing his weapon as if about to knock down an elephant—and fear may be replaced by courage. If the kindergarten teacher who feels disgust at a dirty misshapen baby whose face is covered with sores and pimples will treat him just as she would a dainty, red-cheeked picture of health and clean-

200 *The Principles of Teaching*

liness, take him on her lap, pet him, smile at him and caress him, she will often find disgust giving way to tolerance and even to affection.

This last is indeed the surest way to secure the presence of an emotion. In the long run our feelings grow into harmony with our conduct. Greed cannot live unsupported by greedy acts; the manifestation of love begets it; get pupils to act as they would if the emotion was felt and they will feel it, or, if they do not, will not need to. For in any case they will have the really valuable feature of the emotion, its influence on conduct.

The function of emotions should be to rest and recreate body and mind or to impel to and invigorate thought and action. To merely feel an emotion for its own sake is always a luxury and often a vice. For children to love their native land should mean to study its history; to admire a hero should mean to defend the smaller child and give justice to one's comrades. The majority of the real emotions do not rest body and mind. On the contrary some of them are our most fatiguing experiences. So in general the real emotions should be aroused only for the sake of action. With the aesthetic or pseudo-emotions the practical question is more complicated and unsettled.

§ 46. *The Aesthetic Emotions*

The two questions, 'What is the use of the emotions children feel in reading a story or looking at a picture or hearing music?' and, 'What sorts of emotions should be encouraged in such situations?' will produce various answers from students of education or students of psychology or critics of the arts. Indeed there would be

Responses of Feeling 201

little agreement amongst opinions about what children *do* feel in reading stories and the like.

The commonest opinion among teachers is that the emotions aroused by the arts have a moral value and that the poem or picture should arouse an emotion closely resembling the corresponding real emotion. Such teachers encourage children to talk about a story as if it were a series of real events, to express their opinions of the characters as if they were residents of the next town. If the work of art involves any human or animal actions or conditions such teachers seek to arouse esteem, love, pity, indignation and other such social emotions by it; if it involves only descriptions of inanimate nature they still aim at securing from it feelings of approval, disapproval, peace, joy and the like; even in the case of music, they are tempted to such comments and questions as: 'That makes you feel sad and earnest, doesn't it? This ought to make every boy and girl feel like working. Now we will sing something that will make everybody feel merry and gay.'

Popular opinion takes much the same view as this, but as a rule sets aside certain works of art as simply recreative, useful only as innocent pleasure.

Many of the expert critics of literature, painting and music reject this view as intolerable. To ask a use for art is insulting; it is its own excuse for being, they say. When asked if this means any more than that it gives refined pleasure, they may even assert that it should be studied even if it gave pain to everybody. They would generally stop short of this extreme, however, and admit that it did serve the function of giving a very noble and specially to be desired form of pleasure. Of course, from this point of view the emotion felt toward works of art should be pure appreciation, a response to the aesthetic quality, not any-

202   *The Principles of Teaching*

thing like the emotions which the corresponding real facts should arouse.

From the point of view of the psychologist the facts are lacking from which to draw conclusions about the kind of feelings which children *do have* in connection with works of art, the kind they *ought to be taught to have*, or the value which these feelings would possess. So far as the facts do go, there seems no good reason why children should not be taught to feel something like real sympathy on reading a story of courageous suffering, provided it does not dull or misdirect their real sympathies. On the other hand there seems no good reason why children should not enjoy a story merely as a story, a picture merely as a picture or music merely as music, provided such mental play does not interfere with the business of life. It seems too Puritanical to insist that a work of art should produce pseudo-moral emotions and too artificial to expect specific emotions of any kind to come often from music or always from literature. On the other hand it seems equally artificial to restrict children to mere general aesthetic feeling, whether in the crude form of recreative interest or in the sublimated form of appreciation of art for art's sake.

The test of methods of arousing and guiding the aesthetic emotions is in any case not so much the kind of feeling secured as the use to which it is put. That is good teaching of art which makes it either a stimulus to better conduct or a means of noble, because impersonal pleasure. Just how the teaching secures these results is more or less a matter of indifference.

§ 47. *Exercises*

1. Illustrate the inhibition of the emotion of envy by disuse. By positive repression.

Responses of Feeling 203

2. How would you make use of the method of substitution to get rid of the emotion of rage?

3. Is argument or distraction commonly the better cure for an undesirable emotional condition in a young child? Why?

4. What experience is necessary before a child can be expected to feel awe from reading the burial service?

5. Give two or more illustrations of the law that how anyone feels toward any situation depends upon how he has felt in the past toward that situation or toward situations like it.

6. (a) What emotions do we wish to have felt by ten-year-olds as responses to Christmas day? (b) Which of them are aroused by receiving presents? (c) By giving presents? (d) Why is Dickens' Christmas Carol a good story to read at Christmas?

7. (a) What emotions do we wish boys and girls in the North to feel toward the people of the South and boys and girls in the South to feel toward the people of the North? (b) What was the effect of the history textbook you yourself studied?

8. (a) From the point of view of the emotions what was one advantage of the Puritan way of keeping the Sabbath? (b) What was one marked disadvantage?

9. Why would it be unwise to begin the study of physiology in a high school by exhibiting a skeleton or dissecting a cat?

10. What is the advantage from the point of view of this chapter of making a child's first week in school a week of games, stories read by the teacher, kind words, cheerful occupations and the like?

11. What physical training would you give to cure and prevent the emotions of nervousness and worry?

12. Which of the three methods of securing an emo-

204 The Principles of Teaching

tion is illustrated in the case of the emotion of love for animals on the part of six-year-old pupils by each of these procedures?—

a. Having them read poems such as Stevenson's

The friendly cow all red and white,
I love with all my heart:
She gives me cream with all her might,
To eat with apple-tart.

b. Having some of the children bring their pets to school and care for them there.

c. Having at school pets, rabbits, gold fish, canaries and the like, for which all the class care.

13. Illustrate each of the three methods in the case of teaching loyalty to one's school.

14. What is the value of religious ceremonials, such as kneeling, bending the head and preserving silence in church, in cultivating the religious emotions?

15. Which is the more likely to arouse the feeling that the money power is committing atrocious crimes against the laboring man, hearing A or hearing B? Why?

A. Thou shalt not press down the instruments of torture upon the brow of labor; thou shalt not hang mankind by a halter of gold.

B. Thou shalt not press down the crown of thorns upon the brow of labor; thou shalt not crucify mankind upon a cross of gold.

16. What feeling would probably be aroused by hearing C? Why?

C. Thou shalt not press down a circlet of carpet tacks upon the brow of labor; thou shalt not poison mankind by overdoses of gold chloride.

17. Give one or more illustrations from teaching of the law that to arouse any emotion we should arouse ideas which have gone with that emotion?

Responses of Feeling

18. Give one or two illustrations of mistakes made in teaching by putting together a fact and a feeling which ought to be kept apart.

For Further Reading

A. Bain, *Education as a Science,* pp. 51-112 and Chapter XIII.
W. James, *Talks to Teachers on Psychology,* pp. 199-228.

CHAPTER XIII

MOTOR EXPRESSION

Preparatory, *Elements of Psychology,* §§ 21-22, 25-27, 58

§ 48. *The Relation of Motor Responses to Thought and Feeling*

The Need of Motor Responses.—General psychology teaches that the function of mental life is to modify our bodily responses so as to fit them to the environment and secure life, satisfaction and efficiency. Only in so far as a man's education produces changes in his actual motor responses does it make him of more value to society as a whole; for men influence other people only through their acts. No information or interest or ideal or habit of thought or feeling has done its work until it issues in conduct, until it does something. Moreover, the motor responses which an individual makes react upon his own intellect and character. Not only is his thought worth nothing to anyone else until it alters his acts; it is also worth little to him. Our own movements are perhaps our greatest educators. At any rate they deserve a place beside the impressions made by the physical world and by the conduct of other human beings.

The older psychology was too exclusively concerned with knowledge, and the traditions of education are one-sided in their neglect of the motor consequences of thought. Education must not assume that with the existence of knowledge, its work is done; it must test its in-

Motor Expression 207

fluence by the increased power to express and use knowledge. Education must arouse, control and improve motor as well as mental responses. The expression of knowledge is the only sure sign of its possession and one of the best means of its increase.

True as is the principle that no act of teaching is complete unless it produces some motor consequences, that there should be 'no impression without expression, no reception without reaction,' it must be interpreted intelligently. Expression there should be, but speech and writing are as truly motor as carving or modeling; a change in the pulse or a 'lump in the throat' is as truly motor as dancing in glee or cheering the flag. The inhibition of movement is often to be preferred above its production. Reaction there should be, but it may come a month or a year after the stimulus; it may not come in the form of one definite act due directly to the stimulus alone, but as a slight modification of behavior due to the indirect action of the stimulus and the cooperation of many stimuli.

The Variety of Motor Responses.—Forms of motor expression are well-nigh countless. Not only the movements of the hands in drawing, painting, modeling, constructing objects and the like; not only the movements of the vocal cords and mouth-parts in articulation, accent and song; but all the finer facial movements which constitute facial expression, every shrug of the shoulders, every alteration in breathing and pulse, the tug of the whole body in athletic exercises, labor and combat, and indeed the unnoticed, if not unknown, movements of muscles in the head and throat which perhaps accompany our most secret thoughts—all must be reckoned with in education. The child who whispers 'yes,' the pupil who keeps his eyes fixed on the teacher, the girl who blushes, the soldier whose heart beats more strongly at the call to

208 The Principles of Teaching

battle, the laborer who swings his hammer, the student who sits motionless so far as gross bodily movements go but with every turn of his thought reflected in tensions in the muscles of eyes and throat—all are fundamentally alike in expressing mental states that are and modifying mental states that will be, through motor responses.

Although all forms of motor expression have the same fundamental relations to mental development, it is convenient for practical purposes to separate off language, spoken and written, from all the other forms. The reasons for this separation are that language is particularly specialized, presenting a marked contrast to the rest, that until recently it had almost a monopoly of school education, and that the present problem of the teacher with respect to motor expression is chiefly to preserve the advantages of expression through words and other language symbols and at the same time to enrich the work of the school by the use of the expressive acts of play, art and industry.

§ 49. *Verbal Expression*

The advantages of expression by words and similar symbols are:

1. Their economy of time.
2. Their convenience.
3. Their special fitness to express and arouse general and abstract ideas and judgments and knowledge of relationships.

Economy of Time.—Language is the only means of expression that approaches thought in quickness. There is hardly an object that cannot be named more quickly than it can be drawn; there is hardly an event that cannot be retold again and again in the time it would take to act it out in pantomime.

Motor Expression 209

Convenience.—The development of the random prattling and noise-making of infants into articulate speech expressing nearly the entire realm of human experience, is one of the greatest triumphs of the human species. One is tempted to think that the human species hit upon the best possible means of expression when one considers its extreme convenience.

Oral speech can be carried on regardless of position, regardless of whether one is at the time using arms and legs vigorously; it requires practically no space and no material but air; it expresses thought to hundreds and thousands at once; it produces little fatigue; it needs no very high degree of muscular control; and requires not a great amount of time in acquisition. Written speech adds permanence of the expression and makes hardly greater demands of space, time and material. Next to words drawing is probably the most convenient means of expression, but consider the appliances and technique required for the graphic expression of even a very simple fact. In such expressive work as a good course in manual training offers, the space, apparatus and technical training demanded become a most important consideration. Verbal expression will always be preeminent in the school as it is in life, because of its tremendous advantage on the side of time, space, material and technique.

Special Uses.—Verbal expression, including technical symbols, is peculiarly adapted to the expression of relationships and general and abstract ideas. The very unlikeness of the expression to the fact expressed which differentiates language from pictorial art gives language the possibility of expressing likeness, cause, condition, concession, and other non-representative aspects of experience as easily as red, blue, apple, pear; of expressing a reference to 40,000,000 or to bravery or square root as

210 The Principles of Teaching

easily as to two, the rescue of a drowning sailor or the division of an apple into halves.

Hardly in any other way could we express such facts as in Latin, the usages of *ut* or *quod,* or in grammar the function of tense and mode, or such abstract judgments as π, is the ratio of the circumference of a circle to its diameter,' or 'Virtue is its own reward.' In the work of the school the meanings of many nouns, verbs, adjectives and adverbs, of most prepositions and conjunctions and of all or nearly all pronouns and auxiliary verbs, the logic of arithmetic, grammar (of English and foreign languages), algebra and geometry, the general laws of geography and other sciences and the facts of literature and history that concern human motives and moral values are best expressed in words or symbols for words.

§ 50. *The Activities of the Arts and Industries*

The advantages of expression by constructive and art activities are:

1. Vigor, emphasis, life.

2. Freedom from ambiguity, honesty.

3. Power to express details of shape, color and arrangement.

4. Appeal to interests in action, manipulation and the concrete.

Reality.— Words and figures lack the vividness and emphasis of pictures, models and other material constructions. They do not so easily stir the emotions or so strongly reinforce the original experience of the object. The boy who says, 'A bay is a body of water partly surrounded by land,' makes little impression on others and probably adds less to the clearness and permanence of

Motor Expression 211

his own ideas than the boy who makes a bay in the mud puddle behind the school.

Honesty.—Construction and art are also more likely to be honest, to tell a clear story of knowledge or ignorance. The boy may define the bay from rote memory and yet not be able to recognize a bay if he should see it or to realize its uses. The repetition of words may express real knowledge or only knowledge of words. The pupil himself also realizes the inadequacy of his knowledge of a fact more fully when he tries to express it in a drawing or model than when he answers questions about it. All expression teaches the pupil as well as the teacher, but the constructive act does so in general better than the verbal.

Special Uses.—In many cases words are relatively powerless. The facts concerning the mouth parts of a beetle, the location and direction of rivers, the colors of butterflies or the structure of an engine, can only clumsily and inaccurately and inconveniently be expressed in words; their natural handling is through diagrams and drawings. This is commonly the case with facts of shape, proportion, position and color and is often the case with facts of size.

Interest.— With the introduction into the school of the constructive and art activities, there is a great increment of motive power and zeal from the instinctive interests in the concrete and objective, and in the manipulation of physical things. To write out one's ideas in words is more interesting than to repress them, but the motor process of writing is artificial and difficult and the black marks are so lifeless, so abstract, so remote from the real world that compared with the other means of expression writing is a dull affair. Oral language is more attractive because less artificial and more associated in experience with interesting acts and events; but drawing pictures,

212 *The Principles of Teaching*

working in sand or clay, acting a part in pantomime and the like, rank far higher in the scale of interest. The instincts for action, movement, possession, are behind them, and they do not presuppose the capacity for apprehending the abstract.

Since all the forms of motor expression are useful for mental development, it is the privilege of the school to make use of whatever forms best serve its purposes. The monopoly which verbal expression has so long enjoyed should disappear. The sand pile as well as the slate can record thought. A class in geography should recite with chalk and paint brush as well as with lips. Arithmetic should mean measurement and diagraming as well as calculating. To make a pair of scales is often better than to answer questions about the principles of the balance.

§ 51. *Dangers to Be Avoided*

The dangers in the use of verbal expression are: (1) that the pupils' spoken or written words represent only rote memory or, at the most, a misty, inadequate notion; and (2) that more useful and appropriate motor arts may be neglected.

The dangers in the use of drawing, modeling, constructive work and the like are: (1) triviality, the expression of what is not worth while, (2) the expression of the wrong thing, (3) over-emphasis and misapplication of technique, and (4) injustice to those pupils who have the experience of thought or feeling in question but lack the technique to express it.

Triviality.— There is a great risk that what is drawn, modeled, carved or woven will be from the standpoint of real intellectual advance non-essential. Four hours spent in weaving a red and blue blanket may be worth while as

Motor Expression 213

motor training but they express only a trifle of appreciation of Indian industry and art. The group of pupils who at great expense of time constructed an elaborate cohort of gaily-colored clay knights on horseback may have been well occupied as artists, but so far as concerns real understanding of and feeling toward the activities of the medieval warrior they almost wasted their time. It is not enough to express something; it must be something worth expressing.

Falsehood.—A still worse error is to mistake the expression of one thing for that of something quite different. A teacher who took the square inches of blanket as a proof of appreciation of Indian life or fancied that the table full of colored clay figures witnessed a real understanding of the age of chivalry would probably deceive herself and mislead her class. These constructions probably express ideas of the color and fashion of blankets and of the dress and armor of the knight, and may express only remembrance of certain copies seen. An elaborate drawing of a rabbit may be made by a student utterly ignorant of the essential facts of its anatomy. It is not enough to express something; it must be the right thing.

Over-technique.—It is a constant temptation to emphasize the workmanship at the expense of the story told by any art construction. The student is encouraged to spend hours in drawing a sea-urchin, putting in spine by spine with extreme care, when a rough sketch would answer the purpose nearly, if not quite, as well. Children are allowed or even required to spend all their spare time for a week at coloring in each state on a map, mixing the colors with the utmost care, making all of each state of exactly the same hue and beginning all over if a drop of New York's green happens to spill on Massachusetts. Technical skill is a desirable thing, but it must not be al-

214   The Principles of Teaching

lowed to appropriate time that belongs to motor expression.

Injustice.—Almost everyone has control of the technique necessary to say and write with ease such words as he knows. But many months of study are required to master the means of presenting objects in perspective or of modeling a fair likeness of the human face in clay or of matching a given color with paints. Lack of capacity and training prevents many boys and girls from ever doing justice to their knowledge and emotions in drawing, painting and constructive art. Their technique never catches up with their insight; their art is never equal to their emotions.

Principles of guidance in the choice of means of ex·pression are necessarily somewhat vague: the question is almost always one of balancing advantages and disadvantages. Sometimes the choice is fairly sure; *e. g.,* a drawing rather than words to express the structure of the eye, words rather than a model to express the uses of the Latin word *ut,* a model rather than a line-drawing to express the relation of the earth's orbit to the sun. Sometimes it is difficult; *e. g.,* making maps in relief with sand or flat on paper, speech *versus* drawing and painting in the case of history. The teacher will get on best without fixed rules, keeping in mind the facts of §§ 48-51 and guarding against:

1. Being over-influenced by the convenience of words.

2. Being over-influenced by the attractiveness of manual construction.

3. Relying on words alone to express facts of size, shape, proportion or color.

Motor Expression 215

4. Relying on words, drawing and painting alone to express facts of action and change.

5. Confusing two different things, (a) construction for the sake of motor skill, power over technique and (b) construction for the sake of general mental development.

§ 52. *Exercises*

1. Make a list of ten facts which cannot profitably be expressed in pictures, models or the like.

2. Make a list of five facts which cannot be so expressed at all.

3. Make a list of ten facts which cannot profitably be expressed in words or other abstract symbols.

4. Make a list of five facts which cannot be so expressed at all.

5. Can a pupil express feeling and thought by silence?

6. Clearness, vividness, accuracy, completeness, convenience, economy of time, permanent effect and intrinsic value are the qualities desirable in any means of expression. (a) Which of them are possessed in high degree by drawings? (b) By models made? (c) By schematic diagrams? (d) By spoken words? (e) By gestures? (f) By written words?

7. (a) In which years of school life is the interest in action strongest?

(b) In which years is the appreciation of abstract symbols least?

(c) In which years will the constructive arts be relatively the most valuable means of expression?

8. Give an illustration of the wise use of each of the following means of expression:

a. Pantomime.

b. Writing on a typewriter.
c. Setting type and printing.
d. Measuring.

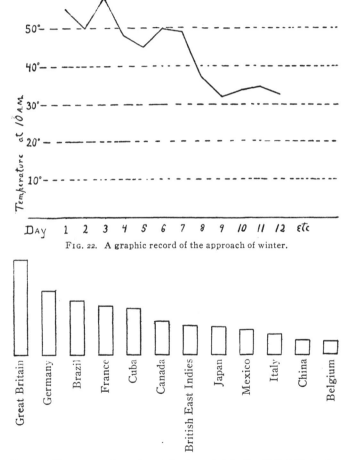

FIG. 22. A graphic record of the approach of winter.

FIG. 23. The comparative value of the imports into the United States from different countries.

Motor Expression

    e. Weighing.
    f. Cooking.
    g. Digging.
    h. Paper folding.
    i. Making 'graphs' such as are shown in FIGS. 22 and 23 (or FIGS. 3-8).
    j. Making machines.

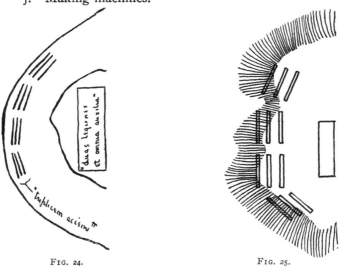

FIG. 24.   FIG. 25.

    9. Illustrate the wise use of drawing as a means of expression in connection with reading, history, physiology, arithmetic, algebra and Latin.

    10. In which cases is it hardest to find a use for it? Why?

    11. Illustrate the wise use of map-making in arithmetic, history and biology or nature-study.

    12. Which was the better teaching, that which secured drawings like FIG. 24 or that which secured drawings like FIG. 25 as expressions of knowledge of the meaning of the following?

218 *The Principles of Teaching*

'Ipse interim in colle medio triplicem aciem instruxit legionum quattuor veteranarum; sed in summo jugo duos legiones quas in Gallia citeriore proxime conscripserat et omnia auxilia conlocari......iussit.'

For Further Reading

W. James, *Talks to Teachers on Psychology*, Chapters III-V inclusive.

J. Dewey, *The School and Society*, Chapters I and II.

E. A. Kirkpatrick, *Fundamentals of Child Study*, Chapter XIII.

CHAPTER XIV

MOTOR EDUCATION

Preparatory, *Elements of Psychology,* §§ 56-57

§ 53. *Teaching Form*

Motor responses as a means of expression of thoughts and feelings were discussed in Chapter XIII. Motor responses as ends in themselves will be the topic of the present chapter. Pronunciation, hand-writing, drawing, singing, painting, modeling and hand work of all sorts involve the existence of connections between certain stimuli and certain movements of the muscles: to learn these acts is to form these connections. The special principles of teaching these acts are, then, principles derived from the psychology of connections of motor skill.

Form and Execution.— Any act of skill is due to two factors,—*form* and *execution.* An individual's form includes whatever he can do deliberately to influence the movement. Thus taking long breaths between sentences, holding the arm and pen in a certain position, making use of certain ways of representing perspective, and recalling that by mixing brown and pink a certain shade can be obtained are matters of form. Execution includes what an individual does without conscious decision because certain movements have been connected directly, not via any intellectual processes, with certain stimuli. Thus giving a certain tone-color to spoken words, speed in writing and

220 *The Principles of Teaching*

the movements of the brush which give a certain curve are matters of execution.

Form concerns associations in which there is an element of thought the connection of which with the appropriate movements is easy to make or already made by previous experience; the problem is to get the right idea. Execution concerns associations in which there is little or no element of thought, the connections being between situation and movement direct; the problem is to get the right connection. If it is already made by previous experience there is no problem at all; the skill has already been acquired.

General Principles.—The principles of teaching form are those of intellectual education generally, modified to meet certain special facts. The pupil needs to be interested in the work, to attend to the instructions and examples given, to understand and remember directions, to be given practice in following them and to be rewarded when he does; explanation, example and drill must all be suited to his natural tendencies and previous experience. The chief modifications are three. Two of these are due to the fact that the idea to be gained is usually one of a complex position of some part of the body. Hence, example is usually far better than rule, imitation more effective than explanation, and the formation of abstractions is rarely necessary or useful. Only concrete thinking about the particular things is required. The third modification is due to the fact that the things to be put together are certain ideas and certain muscular acts, and that consequently the essential thing is what the pupil *does*. Learning how to hold the pen must include actually holding the pen.

Two Dangers.—The chief danger in teaching form is neglect of imitation. There are so many things in school

Motor Education 221

work which need explanation that a teacher gets used to explaining everything. But young children rarely, if ever, learn well such things as how to hold a pen or to cut or to sew by being told how; they have to be shown how. This does not mean that understanding what they are to do or even why that is the best way to do it, is not valuable. It is valuable for pupils to learn to follow directions about technique such as are given in books; *e. g.,* to comprehend why a certain position is taken in planing, or why deep breaths are an essential of good form in running or singing. But such learning is valuable more for the knowledge it gives than for its direct influence in improving form. Imitation of a concrete model is necessary to that end, at least with the majority of pupils.

A second danger in teaching form is to exaggerate the importance of some particular way of doing a thing and so to spend much of the time and effort that ought to be given to concrete execution in insistence upon rigid adherence to some method. If we knew the one best way to write, the one right way to sing and the like, the devotion of much time to form could well be pardoned. But in fact the way a child takes of his own initiative may be nearly as good a way for him as the method his teacher devotes weeks to enforcing. A moderate skepticism about methods of securing proper form in motor accomplishments is healthy. As in reasoning many differing processes may all reach the same conclusion, so in motor skill many different ways of doing a thing may be equally good, one way being the best for some but another way the best for others.

222   *The Principles of Teaching*

§ 54. *Teaching Execution*

The Principle of Habit Formation.—The principles of teaching execution are those of habit formation in general modified in so far as the peculiar nature of the connections,—connections between situation and movement direct,—requires. The important modification is due to the fact that the teacher is less able than in purely mental connections to put together the things he wishes to have go together. One of the things will always be a change in muscular contraction by the pupil, and to make a person contract a muscle when and as we will is beyond our power. A teacher can, by saying 'Three and four are seven' often enough, make sure of the 'three and four—seven' connection in any ordinary pupil's thought; he can put the things together in the pupil's mind, by putting them together as stimuli to the pupil's sense organs. But to make sure of the connection, 'a certain sign on a page—singing a tone a certain exact interval above another,' there is no such easy way. All that can be done to 'put together what ought to go together' is (1) to teach the necessary form and (2) to so arrange circumstances as to increase more or less the probability that the pupil will supply the desired movement.

'To so arrange circumstances' may mean many things. Providing a copy in light ink to be traced over (in writing) and taking pains that only correct models are heard (in the case of the pronunciation of a foreign language) are samples of the ways in which we try to *predispose beforehand* to the right act.

All such are probably of little avail, in comparison with the influence of *selection afterward*. Execution is learned in the main by the 'try, try again' method, by the gradual selection of the successful tendency in consequence of the

Motor Education 223

satisfaction it brings. Execution is taught not by so arranging things beforehand that the right contractions are made, but by stimulating the pupil to many trials and selecting in the course of practice those which are nearest right. *Reward good impulses* is here the prime law of teaching. Even such methods as the tracing and the repetition of the model to be imitated probably possess more influence as selective than as impelling agencies. The letters in light ink tell the child when he moves his pen correctly and make him feel pleased, and conversely: the correct pronunciation remains in memory to rebuke our failures and to reward our chance successes with satisfaction.

In teaching execution then the vital principles are: (1) fitness to capacity, (2) interest, (3) abundant practice directed by proper instruction in form, and (4) the rewarding of good tendencies.

Delayed Motor Capacities.— The capacity to make precise movements matures gradually. Many movements which would be easy for a sixteen-year-old are hard or even impossible for a six-year-old. The latter can, for instance, copy a word written on the blackboard when he cannot copy the same word on a sheet of paper with a pencil. The capacity to make the movements of arm and wrist needed in the former case is not so long delayed as the capacity to make the movements of wrist and fingers needed in the latter. A child who can learn to drive a nail may be unable to learn to thread a needle.

The execution of the movements of writing with pen or pencil, of drawing from a copy, of sewing with an ordinary sized needle, and of moving the eyes in reading from the ordinary primer is of course possible for children in the first two years of school, but it is of the order of difficulty for them that ruling lines one-fortieth of an

224 *The Principles of Teaching*

inch apart or threading needles or reading a book badly printed in Old English type would be for us. It is a form of cruelty, necessary perhaps, to impose such tasks on all six and seven-year-olds. If other things are anywhere nearly equal, blackboard writing, free drawing, telling a story with chalk or pencil and training in making large objects requiring no great exactitude should be substituted, and the reading books should be printed to fit the children, not the traditions of composing rooms. Such changes would save precious time and effort.

Apperception and Execution.—The application of the principle of apperception to teaching motor skill would seem to require that simple elementary movements be taught first and that the more complex ones be acquired as combinations of the simpler. It would seem, for example, that to learn to draw a ship one should learn first to draw straight lines, perpendiculars and simple curves, then to make simple shading to represent solidity, and so on;—that to sing one should get control of single notes, then of simple series of notes, scales and the like, then of total melodies. Plausible as this seems, it is perhaps not the only or the best way to apply the principle of apperception. And it is certainly not the best way to teach children the motor arts. For, even if it gained much by systematically utilizing previous experience, it would lose more from its lack of interest and its failure to form connections in the way that they would later be used.

A motor act for which no present use or bearing is seen, such as singing a solitary note over and over, or writing such exercises as are shown in Fig. 26, or drawing lines that express no fact of moment, can arouse little interest. And since the notes are to be used always in songs, the curves be written always in words and sentences, the lines to be drawn always in a picture of something, it is safe to follow the law of habit formation and so make them from the start. It is risky to put things

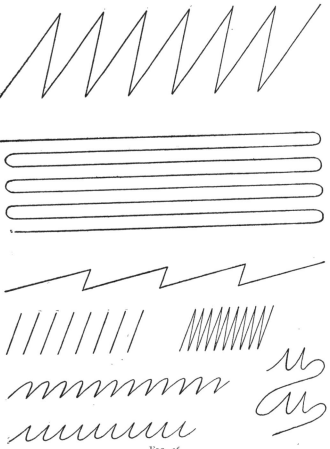

FIG. 26,

together in ways in which they will never have to go together later.

It is by no means sure that the principle of apperception by itself alone does recommend teaching the elementary movements before the complexes apparently made up of them. For the complexes may not be the simple sum of so many elementary movements. Drawing a circle is in fact not the same as drawing a dozen arcs of it, but involves very different movements; writing Fig. 27 is not the same as writing Fig. 28.

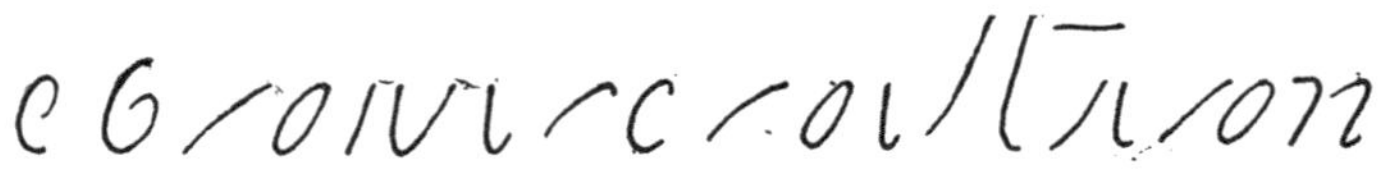

Fig. 27.

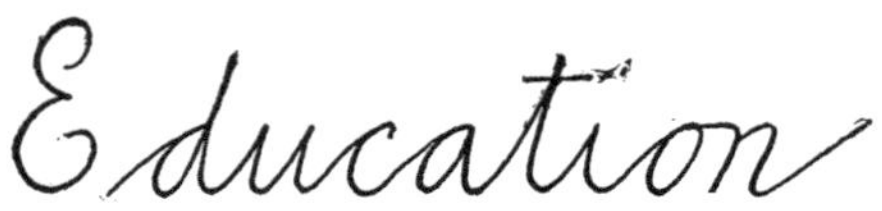

Fig. 28.

Attention and Execution.—Given a general interest in acquiring skill, in doing the thing in hand well, and the less attention to the movements themselves, the better. The facts to be attended to are the guiding sensations, chiefly those due to the changes in the thing that is being made. The penman, that is, should attend, so far as execution goes, not to his fingers but to the words he writes; the singer should, so far as execution goes, attend not so much to the feelings in her throat and chest as to the quality of the tone produced; the worker should attend not to his arm but to the nail that he is driving in. Attend to the situation and the result; the movement will attend to itself.

Teaching Scholars Self-Criticism.—Rewarding good impulses in motor performances is in one way much harder than in the case of mental habits and in another way much easier. It is harder because the good and bad tendencies are in the case of any act very numerous and

Motor Education 227

varied and hence each individual may need approval for a different excellence. In the case of most mental connections there are only a few ways—sometimes only one—of being right, and not very many common ways of being wrong. In a minute or two a teacher may let all pupils of even a large class feel with respect to their answers 'I am right—good!' or 'I am wrong—bad!' But in the case of connections of motor skill a teacher must as a rule inspect each individual piece of work, stamping in desirable tendencies by appropriate treatment of pupils one at a time.

To reward good impulses in motor training is easier in so far as the success and failure of his work is clearer and more emphatic to the pupil than it is in the case of purely mental connections. Children who cannot see that their ideas about geography or history are silly, illogical or mistaken in fact, may see very well that their handwriting is shaky, that there are blots of ink on the page, that the table legs they have made do not fit into the table top. It is easier to tell whether you have made a right angle correctly than whether you have defined it correctly. One can thus learn a trade by himself more easily than a science.

It is wisdom in teaching the motor arts to make this advantage counterbalance the disadvantage of lack of uniformity in product by teaching pupils from the start to be in part their own critics,—to themselves feel satisfaction and discomfort at the right times with less and less aid from the teacher. The teacher's 'This is right: that is bad,' should soon become, 'Which is right? What is bad about that drawing? What do you wish to change in this? Why isn't that just the way you would like it to be?' When good taste is added to strong interest exe-

228 *The Principles of Teaching*

cution will progress rapidly to the limits of the pupil's capacity.

SUMMARY

Teaching motor arts comprises teaching ·form and teaching execution. Good teaching is catholic in permit· ting variations in form, distrusts explanation unassisted by imitation and tests knowledge of form not by questions about it but by its use in actual performance. Good teaching adapts instruction to the gradual growth of motor capacity, forms habits of execution in the way in which they will be used, and makes its chief aims interest and the rewarding of desirable tendencies, first by the teacher but as early as possible by the pupil's own taste and judgment.

§ 55. *Exercises*

1. Which of the following recommendations about teaching penmanship refer to form? Which to execution?

a. "That the left hand rest firmly on the paper." [66]

b. "That the pen be held loosely in the right hand." [66]

c. "That the pupils be taught to criticise the size, slant and space of each letter." [66]

d. "Each slate should be carefully examined by the teacher, and commendation bestowed or corrections made as occasion may require." [67]

e. "If in the course of a writing lesson a child should make several errors of different kinds, it will be better to notice the most prominent first. Too many corrections will tend to confuse the scholar; they should therefore be made one at a time. The teacher should make sure that the child knows exactly what mistake it has made; and for this purpose it will be necessary to speak distinctly and plainly, but not in a fault-finding tone." [68]

f. "Some teachers make a rule that when the children

Motor Education 229

are writing in copy-books the whole class shall write one line in a certain fixed time, say five minutes; that is, that all must begin a line together, and may take the allotted time to complete it; but if the copy should be finished within the time, the next line must not be begun until the teacher gives the command for all to begin the second line. Under such a system much of the time of the more forward scholars will be wasted, and the careless ones who hurry over their work will not be made more painstaking. When simultaneous lessons are being given, especially in the junior classes, this plan is the only one, however, that can be adopted; but when the children are writing independently, no such restriction should be placed upon them." [69]

g. "The Small Letter, i. The teacher opens a copy-book at the page containing the subject of the lesson, or points to the letter upon Chart No. 1, and explains that the letter i is one space in height, and is regarded as the standard by which the height of other letters is measured. He then proceeds to ask questions upon the general form of the letter, thus:

Q. Does the first curve of this letter join the slanting straight line with an angle, or a turn?

A. With an angle.

Q. Where do they join?

A. At the top.

Q. What kind of a turn is formed at the base?

A. A short turn.

Q. What is the rule for making this turn?

A. It should be made as short as is possible, without stopping the motion of the pen.

Q. What relation does the second curved line bear to the first?

A. It is made upon the same slant, and similar to it.

Q. What finishes the letter i ?

A. The dot.

Q. Where is the dot placed?

A. One space above the straight portion of the letter, and on a line with it.

Q. How should it be made?

230 *The Principles of Teaching*

A. By pressing gently upon the point of the pen as if to begin a downward line, and then removing it quickly.

Q. Are there any heavy or shaded lines in this letter?

A. There are none." [70]

h. "The pleasure experienced in personal improvement is in itself a powerful aid in this direction, but in order that the pupil may be made conscious of his daily progress, and thus be incited to renewed effort, a record should certainly be kept of his standing.

A few moments' time before the close of the exercise, will suffice to record in each book the standing of the pupil for the day. A scale of ten may be adopted, or any other which may be preferred.

The teacher may prefer to keep a monthly record, based upon a careful examination of the books. Honors and rewards are frequently conferred upon pupils, to excite a commendable spirit of emulation, and to inspire them with a desire, not so much to excel others, as to surpass themselves. The faithful practice, and unremitting effort essential to progress in the art of penmanship, while bringing, in a measure, their own reward, still merit honorable notice from the teacher." [71]

i. "Entire classes may soon be trained to work in concert, all the pupils beginning to write at the same moment, and executing the same letter, and portion of a letter simultaneously. They will thus progress from letter to letter, and through words and combinations, with all the order, promptness and precision of military drill.

There may be objections to any system of drill which would retard or increase the movements of a mature writer, yet children, or those first attempting the execution of systematic letters, being unable to approximate to a proper speed and uniformity of pen-motion, require some external aid or guide, which will lead them to movements consistent with the proper formation of letters, and, at the same time, prove no obstacle in the way of their subsequent transition to the speed most easy and natural to each individual.

Some pupils move too rapidly, producing letters irregularly, and very imperfect in form; others write with a slow, indolent motion, making downward lines too heavy,

Motor Education 231

turns too broad, and curves uneven. When all are required to write at a medium and uniform rate of speed, the results are more perfect forms, smoother lines, and more regular spacing. The flirt of the pen in the termination of letters, so often indulged in by pupils of every grade, may thus be fully corrected. The counting being uniform, the motion will correspond to it, and sufficient time will be taken to form every line." [72]

2. What are the two letters directions for writing which are given below?

3. How long does it take you to make sure which they are?

4. What is the general error made by the method of teaching penmanship illustrated by these directions?

"First Class Letters. The type of letters of this class is formed by joining the concave curve (characteristic of the class) upon the left and right of the straight line producing an *angle* at the top and a *turn* at the bottom.

Small—is formed by looping the type by a turn to the left at the top and crossing the first upward curve in the middle as its characteristic.

Small—is formed by prolonging the type to twice its usual height, retracing the prolongation, and crossing it in the middle, as its characteristic." [73]

Experiment 14. Close your eyes and write as well as you can with your left hand (right hand if you use the left ordinarily) some sentence of about eight or ten words. Keep the eyes closed and repeat the writing twenty times without seeing the results. In each case write as well as you can. Number the sheets in order 1 to 21. Then write twenty copies (still with the left hand) with eyes open, in each case writing as well as you can. Number them 22 to 41. In which case did you improve most, in the practice from 1 to 20 or in the practice from 22 to 41? Why?

5. Criticise the following:

"TEACHER. What are you going to do? CLASS.

232   *The Principles of Teaching*

To write. T. What on? C. On the copy-book? T. What on in copy-book? C. On the ruled lines. T. What kind of lines are they? C. Straight lines. T. How many different positions are the ruled lines in? C. Two. T. What are they? C. Horizontal and vertical. T. Which are you going to write on? C. On the horizontal. T. Do you notice any other position of straight lines on the page? C. Yes, the straight lines of the principles are oblique. T. You may call each collection of principles at equal distances a Group. What do the vertical lines divide the page into? C. Into columns. T. What are the vertical lines for? C. To separate the groups. T. What is the relative position of the horizontal lines? C. They are parallel. T. What else do you observe, as to their relative position? C. Two are near together, and then the space between is greater. T. What is that for? C. That we may write between the narrow spaces, and make the principles of the right height. T. Will they be of the right height if you do not make them touch both? C. No, sir. T. Then you must be very careful to attend to this. When principles are joined together to make letters, they are said to be connected; when principles are joined together independently, as in these groups, and when letters are joined together, they are said to be combined. In the copy at the head of the first column, what principle is written? C. The first. T. Is it single or combined? C. Combined. T. Which is the main stroke in the principle? C. The first element. T. How is the combination made? C. By the turn and the connecting line. T. What kind of a join is there? C. The end of the connecting line touches the top of the next principle. T. How far, do you think? C. One-fourth of the height. T. This kind of join is called a connection. What is the first element? C. A straight line. T. What is a connection? C. The joining of a connecting line to a straight line. T. How long is a connection? C. One-fourth. T. Is that a long or a short distance? C. Short. T. Is it longer or shorter than the part of the first element which is not touched? C. Shorter. T. How much shorter? C. One-half. T. How is that? I thought you said just

Motor Education 233

now it was one-fourth. C. Yes, sir, one-fourth of the height of the principle, but you asked, 'How much shorter than the part of the first element not touched?' The first element is three-fourths of the principle, one-fourth is touched, so that twice as much remains untouched. Therefore the part touched is one-half shorter than the part untouched." [74]

6. What would be some of the logical results upon methods of teaching oral reading of the acceptance of the following principle?

"Practical mastery of time, pitch, force quality, slides, etc., can be secured only by making them the outcome of an appreciation of the thought and feeling of that which is to be read.

Definite mechanical rules regarding pitch, pauses, slides, etc., are usually worse than useless. Reading is giving expression to a state of mind; it is not the utterance of a series of sounds suggested by the printed page. The flexibility of voice which characterizes earnest conversation may be taken as the best example of the end to be aimed at in reading." [75]

7. Criticise the following lesson from a Fourth reader for "children from seven to twelve years of age":

ORAL ELEMENTS COMBINED

After the instructor has given a class thorough drill on the preceding tables as arranged, the following exercises will be found of great value, to improve the organs of speech and the voice, as well as to familiarize the student with different combinations of sounds.

As the *fifth* element represented by *a,* and the *third* element of *e,* are always immediately followed by the oral element of *r* in words, the *r* is introduced in like manner in these exercises. Since the *sixth* sound of *a,* when not a syllable by itself, is always immediately followed by the oral element of *f, n,* or *s,* in words, these letters are here employed in the same manner.

234   *The Principles of Teaching*

TONICS AND SUBTONICS

1 ba	2 ba	3 ba	4 ba	5 bar	6 baf	1 be	2 be	3 ber
1 ib	2 ib	1 ob	2 ob	3 ob	2 ub	3 ub	ub	oub
1 da	2 da	3 da	4 da	5 dar	6 das	2 de	2 de	3 der
1 id	2 id	1 od	2 od	3 od	2 ud	3 ud	3 ud	oud
1 ga	2 ga	3 ga	4 ga	5 gar	6 gan	1 ge	2 ge	3 ger
1 ig	2 ig	1 og	2 og	3 og	1 ug	2 ug	3 ug	1 oug

(Seven similar tables follow.) [76]

8. What influence would learning the following have upon the act of reading?

Elocution is the mode of utterance or delivery of anything spoken. It may be *good* or *bad.*

Good elocution, in reading or speaking, is uttering ideas understandingly, correctly, and effectively. It embraces the two general divisions, ORTHOEPY and EXPRESSION.

$$\text{Elocution} \begin{cases} \text{Orthoepy} \\ \text{Expression} \end{cases}$$

ORTHOEPY

ORTHOEPY is the art of correct pronunciation.

It embraces ARTICULATION, SYLLABICATION, and ACCENT. [76]

CHAPTER XV

FORMAL DISCIPLINE

§ 56. *The Superstition of General Training*

The Problem.—The previous sections have considered the particular and definite changes wrought by education. We have studied the means of preserving or eliminating particular instincts and capacities, of forming particular habits of attention, interest, thought and feeling, of helping pupils to acquire particular connections of motor response, of selecting and abstracting particular elements, of guiding pupils in particular inductions and particular deductions. The problem has been always, 'What must be done to get this or that particular response?'

Nothing has been said about the means of making general changes in the capacities and powers of pupils, about improving the memory as a whole, or increasing the general capacity to concentrate the mind on any task, or giving the ability to reason well with any problem or to control the mind in all emergencies.

The problem of how far the particular responses made day by day by pupils improve their mental powers in general is called the problem of the disciplinary value or disciplinary effect of studies, or more briefly, the problem of formal discipline. How far, for instance, does learning to be accurate with numbers make one more accurate in keeping his accounts, in weighing and measur-

235

236 The Principles of Teaching

ing, in telling anecdotes, in judging the characters of his friends? How far does learning to reason out rather than guess at or learn by heart a problem in geometry make one more thoughtful and logical in following political arguments or in choosing a religious creed or in deciding whether it is best for him to get married? How far does the habit of obedience to a teacher in school generate the habit of obedience to parents, laws and the voice of conscience?

The Common View.— A common answer of theorists about human life and education has been that each special mental acquisition, each special form of training, improves directly and equally the general ability. Teachers have believed and acted on the theory that the mind was a collection of faculties or powers—observation, attention, memory, reasoning, will and the like—and that any gain in any faculty was a gain for the faculty as a whole. Improved attention to grammar or Latin would thus mean an improvement of the power to attend to any task.

"The common view is that the words accuracy, quickness, discrimination, memory, observation, attention, concentration, judgment, reasoning, etc., stand for some real and elemental abilities which are the same no matter what material they work upon; that these elemental abilities are altered by special disciplines to a large extent; that they retain those alterations when turned to other fields; that thus in a more or less mysterious way learning to do one thing well will make one do better things that in concrete appearance have absolutely no community with it.

The mind is regarded as a machine of which the different faculties are parts. Experience being thrown in at one end, perception perceives them, discrimination tells them apart, memory retains them and so on. By training

Formal Discipline 237

the machine is made to work more quickly, efficiently and economically with all sorts of experiences. Or, in a still cruder type of thinking, the mind is a storage battery which can be loaded with will power or intellect or judgment, giving the individual 'a surplus of mind to expend.' General names for a host of individual processes such as judgment, precision, concentration are falsely taken to refer to pieces of mental machinery which we can once for all get into working order, or still worse to amounts of some thing which can be stored up in bank to be drawn on at leisure." [77]

The powers of the mind are supposed to work irrespective of the data with which they work. The power of observation is supposed to be uninfluenced by the nature of the fact observed; the power to reason to be uninfluenced by the nature of the problem and data; the power of attention to be capable of direction toward any kind of object. It is even said that improvement of any one will improve all of the mental powers; *e. g.*, that learning to attend to Latin forms will make one not only attend but remember, reason and observe better than he did before.

Its Falsity.—The observation of facts proves this answer to be false. It is clear that learning to attend to the cloth in the loom improves the power to attend to printed words or the anatomy of animals little, if at all; that improving in addition from two hundred to two mistakes per hundred examples does not reduce one's errors in judging character by ninety-nine per cent. of their amount; that gaining the power to resist the temptation to steal has little influence on the power to resist the temptation to over-eat. Improvement in one special power rarely, if ever, means equal improvement in general.

238 *The Principles of Teaching*

§ 57. *The Specialization of Abilities*

The exact extent to which the improvement of any special capacity does improve other capacities than itself can be estimated from two lines of evidence, one concerning the extent to which special capacities are related one to another in the human mind and the other concerning the actual effect of special training on general ability as found by scientific investigations.

Common observation should teach that mental capacities are highly specialized. A man may be a tip-top musician but in other respects an imbecile: he may be a gifted poet, but an ignoramus in music: he may have a wonderful memory for figures and only a mediocre memory for localities, poetry or human faces: school children may reason admirably in science and be below the average in grammar: those very good in drawing may be very poor in dancing.

Careful measurements show that the specialization is even greater than ordinary observation leads one to suppose. For instance those individuals who are the highest ten out of a hundred in the power to judge differences in length accurately are by no means the highest ten in the ability to judge differences in weights accurately. In fact they are not very much above the average. The best ten out of a hundred in observing misspellings in words are not very much better off than the worst ten when we test their ability to observe the shape of objects. Similarly quickness and accuracy in thinking of the sums of numbers by no means implies equal quickness and accuracy in thinking of the opposites of words.

The records given below are samples of many that have been obtained by scientific students of education, all testifying to the complex specialization of human capacities, and the existence of variations in any power accord-. ing to the data with which it works.

Formal Discipline

The ranks for 30 students throughout their college course were as follows:

The ranks for 35 4th grade girls in two mental tests[1] were as follows:

The ranks for 25 high-school boys in discriminating lengths and in discriminating weights were as follows:

Individual	Rank in English	Rank in Latin, French & German
A	1	2
B	2	13
C	3	1
D	4	3
E	5	4
F	6	5
G	7	9
H	8	6
I	9	8
J	10	10
K	11	11
L	12	28
M	13	12
N	14	14
O	15	15
P	16	16
Q	17	17
R	18	18
S	19	20
T	20	24
U	21	30
V	22	25
W	23	19
X	24	21
Y	25	22
Z	26	7
a	27	29
b	28	23
c	29	26
d	30	27

Individual	Rank in observation[1]	Rank in Association[1]
A	1	5
B	2	16
C	3	1
D	4	2
E	5	29
F	6	26
G	7	10
H	8	24
I	9	27
J	10	14
K	11	20
L	12	9
M	13	4
N	14	19
O	15	30
P	16	32
Q	17	17
R	18	11
S	19	7
T	20	35
U	21	13
V	22	3
W	23	33
X	24	25
Y	25	29
Z	26	12
a	27	15
b	28	23
c	29	8
d	30	22
e	31	31
f	32	6
g	33	18
h	34	21
i	35	34

Individual	Rank in accuracy with lengths	Rank in accuracy with weights
A	1	4
B	2	8
C	3	24
D	4	12
E	5	5
F	6	17
G	7	2
H	8	14
I	9	6
J	10	7
K	11	20
L	12	23
M	13	9
N	14	11
O	15	15
P	16	10
Q	17	25
R	18	13
S	19	3
T	20	19
U	21	21
V	22	22
W	23	1
X	24	16
Y	25	18

[1] The two tests were: (1) in quickness and accuracy in observing

240   *The Principles of Teaching*

Many facts such as these prove that the mind is by no means a collection of a few general faculties, observation, attention, memory, reasoning and the like, but is the sum total of countless particular capacities, each of which is to some extent independent of the others,— each of which must to some extent be educated by itself. The task of teaching is not to develop a reasoning faculty, but many special powers of thought about different kinds of facts. It is not to alter our general power of attention, but to build up many particular powers of attending to different kinds of facts.

§ 58. *The Amount of Influence of Special Training*

The only sure way to find out how far special training produces general ability,—how far, that is, a change in one particular power improves others,—is to measure the abilities in question before and after the training in question, making proper allowance for the action of other influences than the training, or to compare people who have had the training with people who have not, but are in other respects like those who have.

Such studies have been made in the case of the powers of sense-discrimination, observation and attention, memory and neatness in school work.

Sense-Discrimination.—Bennett found that young children who at the end of several months of training in discriminating different blues had made great improvement, had improved nearly as much in telling apart different degrees of saturation of other colors, but had improved little if any in telling apart lengths or weights.

A's in a sheet of capital letters, words containing certain combinations of letters and the like, and (2) in quickness and accuracy in thinking of the opposites of words. They may be called tests of (1) observation and (2) of association.

Formal Discipline 241

Woodworth and Thorndike found that adults who by special practice had improved greatly in their accuracy in estimating short lines had made no improvement in their power to estimate long lines; and that adults who were trained in judging the size of surfaces of certain shapes and sizes until they had made a decided improvement, showed only about a third as much improvement with areas of different size and shape.

Observation and Attention.— Gilbert and Fracker and Martin have shown that training in responding quickly to one kind of signal produces much but not equal improvement in the quickness of responses to a different kind of signal. Woodworth and Thorndike found that individuals who by special training had improved their ability to notice words containing e and s by a certain amount, showed in the ability to notice words containing i and t, s and p, c and a, e and r, a and n, l and o, misspelled words and A's, an improvement in speed of only 39 per cent. as much as in the ability specially trained, and in accuracy of only 25 per cent. as much. Training in perceiving English verbs gave a reduction in time of nearly 21 per cent. and in omissions of 70 per cent. The ability to perceive other parts of speech showed a reduction in time of 3 per cent. but an *increase* in omissions of over 100 per cent.

Memory.— Different investigators of the influence of memory-training have reached different results, by reason, probably, of differences in their methods; and there is some difficulty in interpreting their results. But in general it is safe to say that training in learning one sort of facts, say Shakspere's Sonnets, by heart will improve the ability to remember other sorts, such as names, dates, lists of numbers and Bible verses, to nowhere nearly the same degree.

242   *The Principles of Teaching*

Neatness.—The only investigation which has been reported of the influence of school training itself, is that of Dr. Squire, who made thorough and careful observations of the neatness of certain classes in their school work as a whole, then gave in school special attention to training in neatness in arithmetical work until the classes reached a high degree of excellence in that particular, and then made observations as before of the neatness of the other written work. Dr. Bagley reports the result as follows:—

"At the Montana State Normal College careful experiments were undertaken to determine whether the habit of producing neat papers in arithmetic will function with reference to neat written work in other studies; the tests were confined to the intermediate grades. The results are almost startling in their failure to show the slightest improvement in language and spelling papers, although the improvement in the arithmetic papers was noticeable from the very first." [78]

Practical Consequences.—From such investigations as these it seems clear that the disciplinary value of studies has been much exaggerated. The one thing of which a teacher can be sure is the particular information, the particular habits and powers, the particular interests and ideals which his training gives directly; he may fairly expect improvement, but less in amount, in abilities closely like that trained; he may hope for some in more remote abilities, but for less and less and finally for none as the ability has less and less kinship with the one directly trained.

The practical consequences are: First, that it is extremely unsafe to teach anything simply because of its supposed strengthening of attention or memory or reasoning ability or any other mental power; when a teacher can give no other reason for a certain lesson or method of

Formal Discipline 243

teaching than its value as discipline, the lesson or method should be changed. Second, that intelligence and care will be necessary to secure from any subject what disciplinary value it does have; we cannot expect that the mere fact that a certain subject is taught somehow will surely result in securing the disciplinary value which it may have when taught properly.

§ 59. *The Method of Influence of Special Training*

To understand how best to secure what general influence any special training does have, we must learn when and how the improvement of one mental function does increase the efficiency of other functions. In the present condition of our knowledge, a complete and perfectly definite answer cannot be given to this question, but the following principles are sure enough for it to be wise for teachers to act upon them.

Through Identical Elements.—One mental function or activity improves others in so far as and because they are in part identical with it, because it contains elements common to them. Addition improves multiplication because multiplication is largely addition; knowledge of Latin gives increased ability to learn French because many of the facts learned in the one case are needed in the other. The study of geometry may lead a pupil to be more logical in all respects, for one element of being logical in all respects is to realize that facts can be absolutely proven and to admire and desire this certain and unquestionable sort of demonstration. Earning one's living for three months may make an improvement in self-reliance in general, for the feelings 'I can do something, I have succeeded, I am not an incompetent,' awakened by self-support are one feature of self-reliance in general. Obedience to one

244 *The Principles of Teaching*

master may make an improvement in general obedience by teaching the possibility and desirability of obedience and self-denial. So in Kipling's story, *Captains Courageous,* a spoiled child who falls overboard from an ocean liner and is picked up by a fishing smack is made sensible and obedient forever after by his experience of necessary submission to the rules of life enforced by the Yankee captain.[1]

Of the millions of situations with which life confronts us many are duplicates, many are identical in important features and still more have something or other in common. One business is in part identical with another business; the sciences overlap; the poet and the musician have somewhat the same task; the concrete habits adapted to life in the country are not all useless in the city; the situations of school are not much like those of the factory or farm but they are not totally different; the process of translating a sentence from Choctaw may have some community with the process of choosing a candidate on election day. Where the community is great, the possibility for the use in one process of ability gained in some other process is great; where the identical elements are but a fraction of the whole, the possibility is little.

These identical elements may be in the stuff, the data concerned in the training, or in the attitude, the method taken with it. The former kind may be called *identities of substance* and the latter, *identities of procedure.*

Identity of Substance.—Thus special training in the ability to handle numbers gives an ability useful in many acts of life outside of school classes because of identity of substance, because of the fact that the stuff of the world

---

[1] Such a case is perhaps more like fiction than truth, for as common an event in real life would be that the spoiled child would retain a grudge against the captain of the fishing boat and would work out his spite on his parents also, his last state being worse than his first.

Formal Discipline 245

is so often to be numbered and counted. The data of the scientist, the grocer, the carpenter and the cook are in important features the same as the data of the arithmetic class. So also the ability to speak and write well in class-room exercises in English influences life widely because home life, business and professional work are all in part talking and writing.

The identity is however not so great as the advocates of the disciplinary value of composition and language study would perhaps ask us to believe. To write 'letters to a friend' or 'stories about a day in the country' or 'es-says on the characters in The House of Seven Gables' is not the same thing as to write an efficient business pro-posal, or to keep a physician's record of cases, or to make a captivating advertisement. Nor is the ability to speak in language classes identical with the ability to speak to jurymen in a law court or to persuade voters.

Identity of Procedure.— The habit acquired in a lab-oratory course of looking to see how chemicals do behave, instead of guessing at the matter or learning statements about it out of a book, may make a girl's methods of cook-ing or a boy's methods of manufacturing more scientific because the attitude of distrust of opinion and search for facts may so possess one as to be carried over from the narrower to the wider field. Difficulties in studies may prepare students for the difficulties of the world as a whole by cultivating the attitudes of neglect of discomfort, ideals of accomplishing what one sets out to do, and the feeling of dissatisfaction with failure.

[1] Here again the advocates of the disciplinary value of studies are likely to overestimate the probability of the acquisition of these ex-tremely valuable ideas and ideals of method and attitude, especially by young children. Such *may* come from special discipline with one study or another, but unfortunately they rarely do. The majority of school boys do their laboratory tasks step by step because they are told to ; their ideas of method being not much more than, 'In history

246   *The Principles of Teaching*

The Means of Securing Disciplinary Value.—The practical consequences of these facts about the method by which special disciplines do attain more or less general results, about the *how* of formal discipline, are that to get the most disciplinary value from any study teachers must select those facts for study which have the most elements in common with life as a whole or which develop best ideas and ideals of attitude and methods which will be useful in life as a whole, and must take special pains that these features of general value are really taught. Otherwise, even where formal discipline is a psychological possibility, it may not be a reality of education. In the case of the features of attitude and method, taking special pains that they are taught means in practice requiring their application to varied situations, for we can never be sure that a general idea or ideal or attitude is gained until we test it in application. Moreover in nine school children out of ten the only way that an ideal or attitude does become general is by being derived from and again applied to many different particular cases. To make ideals and attitudes operative in all fields the teacher must give them exercise in at least several fields.

The facts that the mind is so specialized into a multitude of independent capacities that we alter human nature only in small spots, and that any special school training has a much narrower influence upon the mind as a whole than has commonly been supposed may seem discouraging. It may dishearten the teacher to be compelled to think that the gain in power in arithmentic, grammar or translation does not pass over to all other capacities and powers.

you learn out of a book, in chemistry you watch things boil and take notes, in Latin you try things until you get something like it.' The majority of students learn from the difficulty of studies only the special habits, 'I must do this Latin for if I don't I will only have to do more next year; I must do this grammar for if I don't I'll only have to stay after school.'

Formal Discipline 247

There is however, no real cause for discouragement in finding out these facts. There will be as much disciplinary value to studies as there ever was; indeed more, for having found out how little there is and how that little is obtained, teaching is more likely to have general value than it was so long as we trusted that the subjects themselves would in some mysterious way improve the mind as a whole. The really discouraging thing would be for teachers to delude themselves into wrong choices of subject matter and unwise methods on the basis of false notions about the influence of improvement of one mental function upon others.

It is perhaps unfortunate that learning to do one thing well does not make anyone do everything else much better, that the mind does not repay us ten thousand per cent. on our investments of time and labor. But the mind gives just as much interest after we abandon the superstition of formal discipline as it ever did; and the knowledge of what its rate of interest is and of which investments pay the most can be only a cause for encouragement.

At all events, whether or no we get as much general improvement from special training as we might wish, what we do get comes in no other way. Each special task adds its mite to the general store. Intellect and character are strengthened, not by any subtle and easy metamorphosis, but by the establishment of particular ideas and acts under the law of habit. There is no way of becoming self-controlled except by to-day, to-morrow and all the days in each little conflict controlling oneself. There is no possibility of gaining general accuracy and thoroughness except by seeking accuracy in every situation, by trying to be thorough in every task, by being accurate and thorough rather than slip-shod and mediocre whenever the choice is offered. No one becomes honest

248 *The Principles of Teaching*

save by telling the truth, or trustworthy save by fulfilling each obligation he accepts. No one may win the spirit of love and service, who does not day by day and hour by hour do each act of kindness and help which chance puts in his way or his own thoughtfulness can discover. The mind does not give something for nothing. The price of a disciplined intellect and will is eternal vigilance in the formation of habits.

Moreover, if special training does not give large dividends, they are safe ones; if it drives a hard bargain, it at least redeems every promise. No right thought or act is ever without its reward; each present response is a permanent investment for the future; the little things prepare for the great; the gain achieved by a teacher's efforts is never wasted. The only way to become an efficient thinker and a true man is to constantly think efficiently and act manfully, but that way is sure. Habit rules us but it also never fails us. The mind does not give something for nothing, but it never cheats.

SUMMARY

Training the mind means the development of thousands of particular independent capacities, the formation of countless particular habits, for the working of any mental capacity depends upon the concrete data with which it works. Improvement of any one mental function or activity will improve others only in so far as they possess elements common to it also. The amount of identical elements in different mental functions and the amount of general influence from special training are much less than common opinion supposes. The most common and surest source of general improvement of a capacity is to train it in many particular connections.

Do not rely on any general mental improvement as a

Formal Discipline 249

result of your teaching unless you have actual evidence of it. Teach nothing merely because of its disciplinary value, but teach everything so as to get what disciplinary value it does have. Consider in the case of every subject what ideas and habits of attitude and method the subject should develop that will be of general influence. After securing these ideas and habits in the special subject, give abundant practice in applying them to other fields. The price of the acquisition of general power is eternal vigilance in the formation of particular habits. The special training that is of the greatest value in and of itself will commonly also possess sufficient disciplinary value.

§ 60. *Exercises*

1. Give three or four illustrations from your acquaintances or from historical characters of the fact that a high degree of ability in one direction may go with only a moderate degree of ability in some other direction.

2. For what reality does the term 'the power of observation' stand, *i. e.,* of what actual mental facts should the phrase be used? Answer the same question in the case of the 'power of concentration.'

3. Which of these two statements is the truer?—

A. "It has been well said that an educated man has a sharp ax in his hand and an uneducated man a dull one. I should say that the purpose of a college education is to sharpen the ax to its keenest edge." [79]

B. An educated man has a multitude of useful tools and resources and knowledge of where to get more of the same kind. The purpose of a college education is to increase his stock and practice him in the use of each.

4. Which of these two statements is the truer?—

A. "We speak of the 'disciplinary' studies—having in our thought the mathematics of arithmetic, elementary algebra, and geometry, the Greek-Latin texts and gram-

250 *The Principles of Teaching*

mars, the elements of English and of French or German..
..The mind takes fiber, facility, strength, adaptability, certainty of touch from handling them, when the teacher knows his art and their power. The college......should give.....elasticity of faculty and breadth of vision, so that they shall have a surplus of mind to expend." [80]

B. The study of human nature and of the world of physical facts is more likely to fit the mind to succeed with the problems of later life than is the study of languages or of algebra and geometry. For the habits formed in the latter are less closely related to the habits of later life. The college should give a rich store of well selected knowledge, and training in logical methods applied to the important realities of life.

5 Modify the following statements so that they will not be misleading.

"Let us now examine in detail the advantages which a person who has taken the ordinary Bachelor's degree has derived from the study of classics. Aside from the discipline of the will, which comes from any hard work, we find the following: (1) His memory for facts has been strengthened by committing paradigms and learning a new vocabulary. (2) He has been obliged to formulate pretty distinctly a regular system of classified facts— the facts which from the material of the grammar—classified in due form under chapter, section, subsection and so on. This means that he has learned to remember things by their relations—a power which can hardly be acquired without practice in forming or using such classified systems. (3) He has had his judgment broadened and strengthened by constant calls upon it to account for things which cannot be accounted for without its exercise." [81]

"As regards the first point, it may be noted that the pursuit of mathematics gives command of the attention. A successful study increases or creates the power of concentrating the thoughts on a given subject and of separating mixed and tangled ideas. The habits of mind formed by means of this one set of studies soon extend their influence to other studies and to the ordinary pur-

Formal Discipline

suits of life. The man or woman who has been drilled by means of mathematics is the better able to select from a number of possible lines which may be suggested that which is easiest or most direct to attain a desired end." [82]

6. Comment briefly upon each of the following:

The value of the study of German "lies in the scientific study of the language itself, in the consequent training of the reason, of the powers of observation, comparison and synthesis; in short, in the upbuilding and strengthening of the scientific intellect." [83]

"By means of experimental and observational work in science, not only will his attention be excited, the power of observation, previously awakened, much strengthened, and the senses exercised and disciplined, but the very important habit of doing homage to the authority of facts rather than to the authority of men, be initiated." [84]

"The study of the Latin language itself does eminently discipline the faculties and secure to a greater degree than that of the other subjects we have discussed, the formation and growth of those mental qualities which are the best preparatives for the business of life—whether that business is to consist in making fresh mental acquisitions or in directing the powers thus strengthened and matured, to professional or other pursuits." [86]

"In short, the soul is not a mere knife that may be sharpened on any whetstone, and when sharpened may be applied to any purpose—to cut cheese or to excise a cancer. The knife takes character from the whetstone." [87]

[Advantages resulting from the teaching of drawing.] "The visual, mental and manual powers are cultivated in combination, the eye being trained to see clearly and judge accurately, the mind to think, and the hand to record the appearance of the subjects seen, or the conceptions formed in the mind. Facility and skill in handicraft, and delicacy of manipulation, all depend largely upon the extent to which this hand and eye training has been fostered. The inventive and imaginative faculties are stimulated and

252   *The Principles of Teaching*

exercised in design, and the graphic memory is strengthened by practice in memory drawing. The aesthetic judgment is brought into use, the power of discerning beauty, congruity, proportion, symmetry, is made stronger; and the love of the beautiful, inherent more or less in mankind, is greatly increased." [88]

7. Which of these statements is the truer?

A. "Arithmetic, if judiciously taught, forms in the pupil habits of mental attention, argumentative sequence, absolute accuracy, and satisfaction in truth as a result, that do not seem to spring equally from the study of any other subject suitable to this elementary stage of instruction. [89]

B. Mathematics teaches especially the great value of settled and permanent principles of conduct and procedure, and of adhering to such principles even though they may sometimes appear to be leading to undesirable conclusions." [90]

8. Arrange the following statements in the order of their truth:

A. "Since the mind is a unit and the faculties are simple phases or manifestations of its activity, whatever strengthens one faculty indirectly strengthens all the others. The *verbal* memory seems to be an exception to this statement, however, for it may be abnormally cultivated without involving to any profitable extent the other faculties. But only things that are rightly perceived and rightly understood can be *rightly* remembered. Hence whatever develops the acquisitive and assimilative powers will also strengthen memory; and, conversely, rightly strengthening the memory necessitates the developing and training of the other powers." [91]

B. "I....understand by mental discipline the exercise of some faculty of the mind, which results in increasing the power or readiness of that faculty." [92]

C. "The mind, is, on the the contrary, on its dynamic side a machine for making particular reactions to particular situations. It works in great detail, adapting itself to the special data of which it has had experience. The

Formal Discipline 253

word *attention*, for example, can properly mean only the sum total of a lot of particular tendencies to attend to particular sorts of data, and ability to attend can properly mean only the sum total of all the particular abilities and inabilities, each of which may have an efficiency largely irrespective of the efficiencies of the rest." [93]

Experiment 15. Find some old book printed throughout in the same size and style of type. Cut out 40 pages. Take ten of these pages at random and mark on two of them every verb, on two others every noun, on two others every preposition, on two others every adverb, and on two others every pronoun. Work as rapidly and as well as possible. Get some friend to do the same with ten other pages. Record the time taken for each page and preserve the pages, but without examining them.

Then practice yourself for an hour or so a day in marking on page after page every word which contains both a and t. Record the time for each page during the first ten pages and thereafter the time for each five pages. Score also the number of omissions you make on each page. After you have reduced your time to about 80 per cent. of what it was at the beginning and the number of omissions to a half or a fourth of what it was at the beginning, do ten pages, measuring the time for each page.

Then repeat the tests in marking verbs, nouns and so on and have your friend repeat his tests likewise. Count the omissions in the before-training and atter-training tests with parts of speech? How much improvement is there in your case in quickness and in accuracy in the tests with parts of speech? How much in your friend's case? How much in the tests with words containing a and t? So far as this little experiment goes, how much improvement in the observation of the grammatical

254 *The Principles of Teaching*

features of words is brought about by a given amount of improvement in observing their spelling? What is the use of the tests taken by your friend?

Experiment 16. Use the same tests as before and also, before and after the training, five tests of two pages each in marking words containing (1) both e and b, (2) both i and t, (3) both o and n, (4) two e's and (5) both r and n.

For the special training secure some book with many columns of numbers, all of five figures or of six figures or of seven figures.

Let the training be in marking as rapidly as possible every number in which three successive figures make together (*i. e.*, their sum) 15.

9. Which study has the more elements in common with the problems of life itself, English or Latin? Arithmetic of the elementary school or geometry of the high school? Physics or geology? The sciences of human nature or the sciences of physical things?

10. Which study presents most clearly ideals of accuracy and forms most surely habits of accuracy, arithmetic or geography?

11. Suppose the ideas to be equally clear and the special habits equally firmly fixed, in which case would they be the more likely to give accuracy in statements about people, events and objects? Why?

12. Rank in order for their probable improvement of the power to reason well about education the following: Geometry, Physics, Physiology, Psychology.

13. Rank the same subjects in order for the clearness and convenience with which each in its special field trains deductive reasoning.

14. (a) What subject is specially qualified to give an ideal of deductive proof?

(b) What subject is specially qualified to give an ideal of inductive proof?

(c) What subject is specially qualified to give an ideal of open-mindedness?

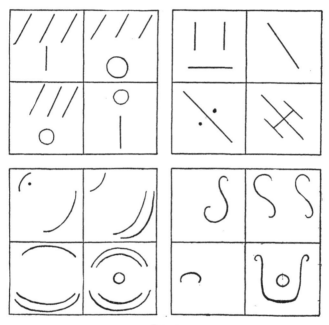

FIG. 29

15. What are the defects of the following as training in observation for children in the third grade: Noting temperature on the thermometer and recording it, and noting the weather and recording it?

16. Would you have a high-school class in biology spend fifteen hours in observing and discussing the external form of a grasshopper? Justify your answer.

17. What means would you take to cultivate the hab-

256 *The Principles of Teaching*

its of open-mindedness and freedom from superstition in nature study in the elementary school or in science courses in the high school?

18. What means would you take to make the habit of open-mindedness about the physical objects studied pass over to the pupil's dealings with all sorts of facts?

19. What criticism would you make of the following method of 'mind-training'?—

Figures like those of FIG. 29 were exposed for a brief time, then removed. The scholars were required to reproduce them. (The figure is a copy of No. 6 of C. Aiken's *Methods of Mind-Training*, p. 48.)

20. Name three or four features of your own school life or that of acquaintances which were due to false notions about mental discipline and which seem to you unjustifiable.

21. Can you think of any mental capacity, to improve which the study of facts in themselves useless is necessary?

For Further Reading

J. Adams, *Herbartian Psychology Applied to Education*, Chapter V.

CHAPTER XVI

THE SCIENTIFIC STUDY OF TEACHING

The efficiency of any profession depends in large measure upon the degree to which it becomes scientific. The profession of teaching will improve (1) in proportion as its members direct their daily work by the scientific spirit and methods, that is by honest, open-minded consideration of facts, by freedom from superstitions, fancies or unverified 'guesses,[1] and (2) in proportion as the leaders in education direct their choices of methods by the results of scientific investigation rather than by general opinion.

Throughout this book the student has been given training in thinking scientifically about teaching, and has been prepared to base his professional work upon facts and to examine every act of teaching in the light of known laws of human nature. One thing more is essential to the proper intellectual attitude of a teacher toward class-room problems—the verification of results.

§ 61. *Testing the Results of Teaching*

The Importance of Tests.— No matter how carefully one tries to follow the right principles of teaching,

---

[1] The right intellectual attitude is, of course, not the sole factor in good teaching. A good will toward children, philanthropic devotion to the work, the zeal for perfection that animates the true artist or craftsman and the personal qualities which work subtly by the force of imitation are also important.

17   257

258 *The Principles of Teaching*

no matter how ingeniously one selects and how adroitly one arranges stimuli, it is advisable to test the result of one's effort,—to make sure that the knowledge or power or tendency expected has really been acquired. Just as the scientist, though he has made his facts as accurate and his argument as logical as he can, still remains unsatisfied until he verifies his conclusion by testing it with new facts, so the teacher, after planning and executing a piece of work as well as he can, must 'verify' his teaching by direct tests of its results and must consider uncertain any result that he cannot thus verify.

Their Difficulty.— It is true that some of the most important results of teaching cannot be verified at all by the teacher himself. The permanence of interests, the effect of moral inspiration in childhood on adult behavior and the fortification of the pupil's heart against degrading forces that will assault it years after school is done, are of necessity not subject to full or accurate verification. The results of a teacher's work upon the life of the pupils out of school are also to a large extent inaccessible to adequate observation. Finally certain changes in human intellect and character, such as nobler ideals, new ambitions and stronger powers, are hard to test even within the sphere of school and class-room life. The deeper ideals and ambitions are often cherished in secret and revealed only by some sudden access of intimacy or by unusual events. The strength of mental powers is not hard to test but the result is almost always the result of delayed capacity,— of mere inner growth,—as well as of the teacher's efforts; hence, the facts are hard to interpret.

In many cases, however, a teacher may not only hope and believe that a desired result has been obtained; he may know. In many cases he can do more than simply try the best plan he can devise; he can try, test the re-

The Scientific Study of Teaching 259

sults, find the failures in them, and, with this new knowledge, devise a remedy. Such actual verification of the success of one's work is possible in the case of changes in knowledge, skill and all definite habits. One should be able to tell absolutely whether Johnny Smith gets ideas or only words when he reads, whether Mary Jones can sew well enough to be worth five dollars a week to a dress-maker, whether Fred Brown does or does not treat his class-mates with more justice than he did three months ago.

Their Value to the Teacher.—Testing the results of one's teaching is useful not only because it gives a basis for improvements in one's methods, but also because it is one chief means of gaining knowledge of the mental content and special capacities of individuals. In applying the principle of apperception a teacher is constantly led to test the results of knowledge previously given as a preliminary to giving more. For the main thing in fitting stimuli to the mental make-up of pupils is not a host of ready-made devices to secure the cooperation of previous experience; it is rather constant readiness in testing for the presence of the essentials, in diagnosing the exact result of previous lessons.

Their Value to the Class.—Testing the results of teaching is useful to the class as well as to the teacher, and to the class directly as well as indirectly through the betterment of future steps in teaching. Any scholar needs to know that he knows as well as to merely know; to be ignorant and know that you are so is far more promising than to be ignorant and not know it. By expression and use new ideas and habits get a double value; boys and girls in school need to know what progress their efforts have achieved and to guide their efforts by objective facts as well as by their own sense of progress.

260   *The Principles of Teaching*

It is a common opinion that examining a pupil, finding out 'whether he knows his lesson' is the least part of teaching, is something that anyone can do.   And it is fashionable amongst many teachers to spend the greater part of their time and still more of their energy in giving children opportunities to learn a great deal rather than in making sure that they learn something.   The type of testing that uses the entire recitation simply to make sure that the pupil has studied certain pages of a book and remembered what he has learned is a small part of teaching and can be done by even a poor teacher.   But the real verification of the work of teaching, that makes sure of just what the pupil knows and feels, that tests his comprehension and attitude as well as his memory, that prevents waste and prepares the way for better teaching of that pupil in the next topic and better teaching of that topic with the next class, is a most essential part of teaching and is one of the hardest things to do well.

The Principles of Effective Testing.—The principle is indeed easy but its successful, concrete application requires both a high degree of capacity for insight into the facts of child life and thorough training.   The principle is simply:—To know whether anyone has a given mental state, see if he can use it;[1] to know whether anyone will make a given response to a certain situation, put him in the situation arranged so that that response and that response alone will produce a certain result and see if that result is produced.   The test for both mental states and mental connections is appropriate action.

[1] This is not given as a principle of psychology or logic, but as a rule for teaching. We are not here concerned with an ultimate criterion for the existence of a mental state in a given individual, but with a practical means of being assured that John has a certain concept of the class 'dog,' that Mary knows what 'seven' means and the like.

The Scientific Study of Teaching 261

The test is easy to apply in the case of responses of bodily action. Can John write his name? Ask him to. Can Mary make edible biscuit? Set her to work and try to eat what she makes. Will John obey the teacher? Give him orders. It is also easy in the case of verbal memory,—for all that is meant by verbal memory is clearly evidenced by the bodily actions of saying the words.

It is harder, but still fairly easy, to apply in the case of connections of impression. That it is not very easy is shown by the fact that teachers often think a child stupid or even refractory when the real fact is that he does not clearly hear, does not get the impression of the questions they ask; also by the fact that a boy may fail in painting or work with colored maps because of color-blindness and receive reprimands from the teacher for supposed lack of attention.

The error is in neglecting the 'that response alone.' The teacher acted on the theory: 'To fail to answer an easy question is the result of perversity or stupidity. This boy fails again and again. To color a map pink in spite of my clear directions to use green is the result of inattention.' A converse error is made by teachers of science who say; 'If a pupil really sees the specimen he can draw it,' and so use the power to draw as a test of the existence of certain responses of perception or observation. They are clearly wrong in the case of seeing things properly in three dimensions and drawing in perspective, and are as truly if not as emphatically wrong in the case of many other features of drawing which make technical demands. Logically it would be as true to say; 'If you see the specimen as it is, you can draw it,' to an armless man as to some students. The error here is of course in supposing that the response will always produce the 'cer-

262 The Principles of Teaching

tain result,' and so inferring the absence of the response from the absence of the result.

The principle is much harder to apply in the case of responses involving the knowledge of the meanings of words, figures and other symbols, comprehension of processes, rules, arguments and the like, appreciation of literature and the arts, feelings for nature and human beings, attitudes of interest and attention and other connections involving purely mental elements.

In such cases it often requires much ingenuity and experimentation to find a result which shall be a sure test of the presence of the response in question. Suppose for example that a teacher wishes to know whether the members of her first-year class in reading respond to the sight of *unless* by a feeling of its meaning. For them to read it correctly tells little or nothing. For them to define it correctly might mean merely verbal memory of a definition. On the other hand they might be unable to define it at all satisfactorily and still know what it meant as well as was necessary. To ask them to give orally and write a sentence with *unless* in it is a step in the right direction, especially if several such sentences are required, but correct use in several sentences is not always a clear symptom of knowledge of meaning, for by purely spontaneous association the word *unless* may call to memory sentences containing it, and occasionally, though very rarely, a child who knows what *unless* means may not think of a sentence that suits him.

To test for knowledge of this one word requires, in fact, a rather complicated procedure, for instance the completion of the following sentences so that they make sense. Success with five out of the eight would be almost certain evidence of sufficient knowledge of *unless* for the purposes of primary reading.

The Scientific Study of Teaching 263

It is dark at night unless............
It is light in the daytime unless............
I like to go outdoors unless............
They cannot read unless............
He will come unless............
He will not come unless............
She would do it unless............
The stove is hot unless............

Testing Knowledge of Terms.— To know what a triangle is, is to be able to recognize one when seen, to be able to pick out all the triangles from a miscellaneous collection of areas, to know where you will arrive at the end of the third side if you walk around it, to know how many sides will be left if you stand it up on one, and the like. With pupils of a certain degree of motor ability and practice with scissors, ruler and pencil, to know what a triangle is will imply ability to draw one, to draw four or five different ones, to cut different shaped triangles out of paper and the like. To recognize, to classify, to answer questions about, to know what to expect of and to construct a thing are all useful and significant as tests of knowledge of it. To define it is simply to try to summarize the answers to possible questions about it. The question, *What is a* — has the advantage of asking many questions in one, and the disadvantages of asking them vaguely and of encouraging the repetition of some set form. When a definition is the result of a pupil's observation or recall of many facts about the thing, of selection of the essential ones and their statement by him, it is a very valuable test of his knowledge.

The general principle for testing the results of teaching may be illustrated further by some of the prohibitions which it implies:—Distrust the repetition of words as a test of anything more than verbal memory.

Use definitions but never as a sole test;—the power to

264　　　*The Principles of Teaching*

define may exist without the knowledge of the term and knowledge of a term may exist without the power to define it.

Distrust any one particular kind of problems as a test of appreciation of a law. Distrust especially problems that are familiar or of a well-known type.

Do not take it for granted that the ability to handle certain elements when isolated implies the ability to handle the same elements in complex connections.

Do not test the ability to do one thing by the ability to do something else if a direct test is practicable.

SUMMARY

Testing the results of teaching and study is for the teacher what verification of theories is to the scientist,— the *sine qua non* of sure progress. It is a chief means to fitting teaching to the previous experience and individual capacities of pupils, and to arousing in them the instinct for achievement and the capacity for self-criticism. The test for knowledge, skill, appreciation and morality is in each case appropriate action. A valid test is one in which the response in question (knowledge or skill or ideal or whatever it may be) and only that response will produce a certain observable result.

§ 62. *Testing the General Results of School Work*

The Importance of Tests of Methods.—What the teacher should do with respect to each act of teaching each pupil, the leaders in education should do with respect to the general methods of teaching a subject recommended to all teachers. Expectations of results, even if based on right principles, must be corroborated by actual verification.

The Scientific Study of Teaching 265

As a rule the best present judgment about the efficiency of a method of teaching will rest upon its harmony with the principles derived from the facts of human nature and upon its success or failure as measured by the opinion of those who try it. The best present judgment will not be mistaken very often or very much, but there could be safer tests of the worth of methods. For when a principle derived from the facts of human nature is applied under the peculiar conditions of school life it may need modification; and the opinions of even the best teachers concerning the value of a method may be shortsighted and partial. What is needed is the comparatively sure decision of that superior variety of opinion which is called science.

The Characteristics of Scientific Judgments of Methods.—The judgments of science are distinguished from the judgments of opinion by being more impartial, more objective, more precise, more subject to verification by any competent observer, and by being made by those who by their nature and training should be better judges.

Science knows or should know no favorites and cares for nothing in its conclusions but their truth. Opinion is often misled by the 'unconscious logic of its hopes and fears,' by prepossessions for or against this or that book or method or result. Science pays no heed to anything but the facts which it has already made sure of; it puts nothing in the scales but objective evidence. Opinion trusts its personal impressions, bows to authority and follows the crowd. Anyone's opinion constantly favors the methods he is used to and is suspicious of new ideas except his own; it accepts without verification and rejects without a fair trial. Science seeks precise quantitative measures of facts by which changes and correspondences

266   *The Principles of Teaching*

may be properly weighed·; opinion is content to guess at amounts of difference and likeness, to talk in the vague terms of more or less, much and little, to rate a method as better or worse without taking the pains to find out just how much better or worse it is. Science reveals the sources of its evidence and the course of its arguments, so that any properly equipped thinker can verify for himself the facts asserted to be true. Opinion offers itself to be accepted or rejected, but not to be verified or intelligently criticised. Science is the work of minds specialized to search after truth and selected as fit for the work by their equals and superiors in it. Opinion is the occasional thought of those who, though important and capable people, are yet only amateurs in the work of getting truth.

Science would decide between two methods, say of teaching reading, by giving each an adequate trial, by measuring exactly the changes in bodily welfare, knowledge, interests, habits, powers and ideals caused by the two, and by comparing impartially the results in the two cases. It would, for instance, arrange that method A should be tried in ten or twenty classes and method B in ten or twenty other classes of equal ability and advantages taught by equally competent teachers. It would make sure that the two groups of teachers tried equally hard and that the two groups of classes were alike with respect to school-room equipment, the amount of time given to reading and the like. It would measure with precision the accomplishment of each pupil in reading itself, in spelling and writing, in knowledge of facts gained, in appreciation of good literature, in interest in reading, in such habits as might be influenced by the special training of reading, in power to learn new things and so on

The Scientific Study of Teaching 267

through the list of all the changes which instruction in reading may produce.

The Prospects of Scientific Investigations of Teaching.— Obviously such a scientific basis for the professional work of teaching is in every way desirable. But for many reasons only a beginning has been made. The main reasons are perhaps, first that strictly scientific methods have only lately begun to be used in the case of facts of human activities and second that the complexity of the problems of teaching is so great as to make scientific treatment of them very intricate and laborious. There are a score of competent scientists engaged in the study of physical science for every one that is at work on the problems of social institutions. The task of knowing completely the facts and explanation of the mental and moral development of any one child is comparable to the study of the geology of an entire continent or the chemistry of all the metals.

The infrequency of the effort to investigate questions of teaching in the spirit and by the methods of science and the difficulty of the task itself are, however, no excuse for their neglect. The scientific study of teaching is at least as important as the scientific study of medicine and, though difficult, is in no way impossible. Even the subtle changes in powers, interests and aspirations can be measured; for sooner or later they must be manifested in actual facts. Even the remote influences of teaching on life after school can be known if the investigator has unlimited time and energy. The immediate influence of various sorts of teaching upon the knowledge and habits directly concerned, may be studied scientifically with much less difficulty and with promise of quick returns in knowledge. There should be no need to guess at the value of methods

268   *The Principles of Teaching*

of teaching spelling or beginning reading or Latin grammar.

Such investigations lie beyond the scope of the activities of most teachers. The time, the training, the scientific frame of mind and the zeal which they require can only rarely be at the disposal of the teacher, who has so many other things to learn and to do. To advance scientific knowledge of education is a most worthy occupation for anyone who is able to succeed in it but it is not the duty of all or of many teachers. The burden of making exact measurements of children's attainments, of inquiring deeply into the what and why of the facts of school life and of feeling responsible for the verification or disproof of hypotheses about methods may be assumed voluntarily by the investigator, but it should not be imposed upon an already too busy teacher. Teachers should respect and encourage the labors of science but they should not feel bound to share them. The leaders in thought about education, on the other hand, *should* feel bound to study scientifically the field in which they claim to rank as experts. Since their opinions will be accepted by the profession as a whole, it is their duty to verify each opinion by a test of the results to which it leads.

§ 63. *A Typical Scientific Study of School Work*

As a sample of what we may expect from scientific tests of the results of teaching I shall summarize and quote from Dr. O. P. Cornman's investigation of the value, or rather, lack of value, of specific drill in spelling.[1]

---

[1] Dr. Cornman's entire investigation (*Spelling in the Elementary School; An Experimental and Statistical Investigation.* Vol. 1 of *Experimental Studies in Psychology and Pedagogy,* from the Psychological Laboratory of the University of Pennsylvania, 1902) deals also with individual and sex differences in spelling ability, the influence of age, grade and general mental capacity and the nature and causation of errors in spelling, his study of the needlessness of special drill in spelling being only one division of the investigation.

The Scientific Study of Teaching 269

Dr. Cornman found first that the ability to spell of one school population as compared with others in the same city showed 'a conspicuous want of correlation' with the amount of time devoted to spelling drill. In this particular he corroborated the results of Dr. J. M. Rice's work. In both cases schools devoting three times as many hours per year to specific spelling instruction as other schools showed little or no superiority in the spelling of their pupils.

The material from which he drew this conclusion consisted of tests of 11 schools made in 1897, of 19 schools made in 1899 and of fifty schools made in 1900. Each school gave results from seven or more classes. A sample of the material is given below.

RECORDS OF 1898

School	4th a grade		5th grade	
	Time given to spelling; minutes per week.	Ability of the class in spelling.	Time given to spelling; minutes per week.	Ability of the class in spelling.
A	50	67.0	50	68.0
C	75	75.5	60	72.5
E	100	76.4	80	83.5
F	100	65.0	100	57.4
G	100	66.0	100	76.2
D	120	65.0	100	66.0
I	150	70.3	100	67.1
H	200	76.3	160	82.0

Dr. Cornman's main experiment was to omit entirely specific drill in spelling from the program of two schools for a period of three years, and to observe the results. He outlines the plan of the experiment as follows:

"The results of the experimental investigation of spelling errors and the psychological facts and theories bearing upon the acquirement of spelling habits, which were given in the preceding section, suggest the comparative meagreness of the contribution of the specific spelling drill to the

270　The Principles of Teaching

final result, and warrant an experiment which might otherwise have seemed a too dangerous tampering with the educational progress of the pupils who were to act as subjects in the tests.

It was decided to abandon the use of the spelling book and home lessons in the subject, to omit also the period from the school programme which had been devoted to its study and recitation, and to investigate the effect that the abstraction of these influences might produce upon the spelling of the pupils of the several school grades. Several methods of measuring results were devised which will be herein described and statistically reported upon." [94]

The results were as follows:

In spite of the omission of specific instruction in spelling, the pupils improved steadily.

The work of the two schools in spelling was nearly or quite as good as in previous years when special drill in spelling had been the rule for every class.

The work of the two schools in spelling was nearly or quite as good as that of other schools in the same city who retained the spelling drill. There was little or no more difference than there had been in previous years.

The sources of the data from which these results were obtained were as follows:

Eight composition tests were given in 1897-1898, 3 in 1898-1899 and 3 in 1899-1900 to all the pupils in the Northwest School (approximately 600) and ten composition tests to all the pupils in the Agnew School (approximately 160).

All the pupils in the Northwest School were also tested at the end of the school years 1895-1896, 1896-1897 and 1897-1898 in writing as many words as they could in 15 minutes, the percentage spelled correctly being computed for each pupil. The papers written in June, 1898, after a

The Scientific Study of Teaching   271

year's omission of spelling drill were compared with those written in June, 1897.

Dr. Cornman also used "the data afforded by the regular term examination in spelling (which is prepared in the office of the superintendent and is the same for all the schools of Philadelphia) to compare the results of the Northwest and Agnew schools with those of other schools pursuing the usual course of specific instruction in spelling." [95]

The spelling work of all pupils of the Northwest and Agnew schools in the examinations of January, 1898, June, 1899, and June, 1900, was recorded, and also the class averages for 11 other schools in the examinations of January, 1898, for 19 other schools in the examinations of June, 1899, and for 50 other schools in the examinations of June, 1900.

All the children of the Northwest and Agnew schools were also tested in June, 1897, and June, 1898, with a list of fifty isolated words and a long list of words to be written in sentences.

Finally four tests each of fifty isolated words were given to all the children of the Northwest and Agnew schools at intervals throughout the year 1898-1899. Each test "consisted of fifty words selected from a 'Review List of Difficult Words' for the particular grade to be tested, found in a modern spelling book. The review words (about five hundred in a list) were arranged in alphabetical order, and the fifty words for the first list were selected by taking the first, fifth, ninth, thirteenth word, etc.; those for the second list, by taking the second, sixth, tenth word, and so on. In this way lists were secured presenting approximately equal degrees of orthographical difficulty." [96]

Dr. Cornman thus had sufficient material to compare

272　The Principles of Teaching

classes who had, for a year or for two years or for three years, no special instruction in spelling with classes of the same grade in other schools and in the same school in previous years, who had had such special instruction. He had sufficient material to compare them both in the spelling ability attained and in the progress made from their condition of a year or two years or three years before. I give the figures for a few of such comparisons.

Spelling ability measured by uniform examinations for all schools, given by the city superintendent.

50 schools giving specific instruction in spelling.		2 schools in which for three years no specific instruction in spelling had been given.
7th grade	73.0	69.9
6th "	70.4	65.1
5th "	71.6	72.7
Average	71.7	69.2

The spelling ability of classes in the Northwest School who had for three years been without specific instruction in spelling compared with that of corresponding grades of previous years, who had had the full amount of drill in spelling.

	Tests of June, 1897.	Tests of June, 1900.
8th grade	99.4	99.8
7th "	99.1	98.6
6th "	96.75	99.0
5th "	96.95	97.6

The spelling ability in a test in writing words in sentences of classes which had been without specific instruction in spelling for a year and of classes which had had regular drill.

	Classes with regular drill. Tests of June, 1897.	Classes without regular drill. Tests of June, 1898.	Difference
Northwest 8th grade	89.8	90.6	+ 0.8
7th "	86.1	78.7	− 2.6
6th a "	83.5	77.5	− 6.0
6th b "	72.7	71.7	− 1.0
5th a "	80.6	76.9	− 3.7
5th b "	78.8	79.2	+ 0.4
4th a "	75.1	80.7	+ 5.6
4th b "	85.8	85.3	− 0.5
3d a "	86.5	70.4	−16.1
3d b "	57.8	57.7	− 0.1

The Scientific Study of Teaching 273

Agnew	4th a grade	76.8	82.0	+ 5.2
	4th b "	82.5	83.7	+ 1.2
	3d a "	72.3	73.7	+ 1.4
	3d b "	66.1	67.7	+ 1.6

That is, half of the classes without specific instruction did better and half of them worse than the corresponding classes with specific instruction.

His facts justify his conclusions that:—

"(6) The amount of time devoted to the specific spelling drill bears no discoverable relation to the result, the latter remaining practically constant after the elimination of the spelling drill from the school programme.

(9) It is therefore advisable, in view of the economy of time, to rely upon the incidental teaching of spelling to produce a sufficiently high average result.

(10) This average result is what *can be* and *is* attained, as shown by statistical evidence, by average pupils under teachers of average professional efficiency in classes of average size, *i. e.,* in the elementary schools of this country as now organized. To remain strictly within the evidence gathered by this investigation, it must be admitted that there *may* be teachers of surpassing ability, who can obtain more than average results by the method of the specific spelling drill, and other teachers of meaner ability who need the drill to bring their pupils up to the level of this average result. It is claimed, however, that there is no evidence (whatever may be the wealth of *opinion*) to *prove* that such teachers exist or to show where they may be found. Moreover, the evidence which has been presented in this paper makes their existence at least improbable." [97]

Topics for Further Study

These topics and the references given with each are chosen to meet the needs of the students who use this book as a text, not the needs of expert students of education. In choosing the references, accessibility, convenience and intelligibility are given as much importance as specific restriction to the topic or excellence from the expert's point of view in treating it. Rare books are rejected; books in foreign languages and articles in periodicals are used rarely or as optional references. Books are given a decided preference over scattered articles, not only because they are so much more accessible and convenient for the student's use, but also because the complete, systematic presentation characteristic of a book is a great advantage to college and normal school students. The list does not aim to be an adequate representation of the topics which may be studied under the heading 'Principles of Teaching.' Indeed it aims precisely to be *not* complete, but a selection such as will make the student's reading more effective. The ten books referred to throughout the text under 'For Further Reading' would of course be included in the present list, had they not been used as collateral reading for the different chapters.

The General Principles of Teaching

1. The Ultimate Aims of Teaching. *The Meaning of Education,* by N. M. Butler, or *Educational Aims and Educational Values,* by P. H. Hanus, or *The Philosophy of Education,* by H. H. Horne.

274

Topics for Further Study 275

2. Physical Education. *Physical Education,* by A. Maclaren.

3. The Hygiene of Reading and Writing. Chapters VII-XI of *School Hygiene,* by E. R. Shaw, (1901) or Chapters I-III, V-VIII, and X-XI of *The Physical Nature of the Child,* by S. H. Rowe (1899).

4. Nervousness and Allied Disorders. *The Study of Children,* by F. Warner.

5. Instinct and Habit throughout Nature. *Habit and Instinct,* by C. L. Morgan.

6. Apperception. *Apperception,* by K. Lange (edited by C. De Garmo).

7. Realities *versus* Words in Teaching. *An Experiment in Education,* by M. R. Alling-Aber and *Object Lessons, or Words and Things,* by T. G. Rooper.

8. Interests. *Interest and Education,* by C. De Garmo and *The Child and the Curriculum,* by J. Dewey; or *Interest as Related to Will* (Second supplement to the Year-Book of the Herbart Society for 1895; second edition, 1903), by J. Dewey and *Interest in its Relation to Pedagogy,* by W. Ostermann (edited by E. R. Shaw).

9. The Correlation of Studies. *Number Work in Nature Study,* by W. S. Jackman.

10. Attention. *The Art of Securing Attention,* by J. G. Fitch and Chapters XII-XVI of *The Art of Study,* by B. A. Hinsdale.

11. Inductive and Deductive Teaching. *The Essentials of Method* (revised edition, 1897, or later), by C. De Garmo.

12. The Influence of School Education upon Conduct. *The Moral Instruction of Children,* by F. Adler, or Pages 1-100 of the *Third Year-Book of the National Herbart Society* (1897), by J. Dewey, C. De Garmo, W. T. Harris and J. Adams.

13. The Importance of Motor Responses. *The Place of Industries in Elementary Education,* by K. E. Dopp (1905 or later).

276 *The Principles of Teaching*

14. The Dogma of Formal Discipline, Chapter XIII of *The Educative Process*, by W. C. Bagley (1905), *The Dogma of Formal Discipline,* by B. A. Hinsdale and Chapters XIII and XIV of *Education as Adjustment,* by M. V. O'Shea (1903).

15. Scientific Investigations of Teaching. *Spelling in the Elementary School,* by O. P. Cornman.

16. Teaching from the Point of View of Psychology. *The Educative Process,* by W. C. Bagley.

17. Teaching from the Point of View of Direct Experience. *Common Sense in Education and Teaching,* by P. A. Barnett, or *Principles of Class Teaching,* (especially sections IV and V) by J. J. Findlay, or *Lectures on Teaching,* by J. G. Fitch, or *Talks on Pedagogics,* by F. W. Parker, or *Elements of Pedagogy* (the division entitled 'Methods of Teaching') by E. E. White.

18. Teaching from the Point of View of Pedagogical Theories. *General Method,* by C. A. McMurry, or *Outlines of Pedagogics* by W. Rein (translated by C. C. and I. J. Van Liew), or *The Philosophy of Teaching,* by A. Tompkins.

19. Teaching Children of the Kindergarten Age. *A Study of the Kindergarten Problem,* by F. and C. F. Burk and *Kindergarten Principles and Practice,* by K. D. Wiggin and N. A. Smith.

20. Teaching in the Primary Grades. *Primary Methods,* by W. N. Hailmann (a book that pretends to treat only one narrow aspect of the problem and hence one that should be read only in connection with other books) and *Nature Study Lessons for Primary Grades,* by L. B. McMurry; or *Physiological Notes on Primary Education,* by M. P. Jacobi and *Special Method in Primary Reading,* by C. A. McMurry.

21. Class Management and Discipline. Chapters III and IV of *School Management and Methods of Instruction,* by G. Collar and C. W. Crook (1900) and Chapters VII-X of *School Management* by S. T. Dutton.

Topics for Further Study 277

22. The Teacher as a Logician. *The Principles of Logic,* by H. A. Aikins or *The Logical Bases of Education,* by J. Welton.

23. The Teacher as a Worker in a System. *Our Schools: Their Administration and Supervision,* by W. E. Chancellor.

24. The Teacher as a Co-worker with Social Forces outside the School. *Democracy and Social Ethics,* by Jane Addams, or *The Principles of Religious Education,* by N. M. Butler, W. C. Doane, C. De Garmo and others, or *Social Phases of Education,* by S. T. Dutton, or *Industrial Education,* by Philip Magnus, or *Poverty,* by R. Hunter and *The Children of the Poor,* by J. A. Riis, or *The Problem of the Children and How the State of Colorado Cares for them: A Report of the Juvenile Court of Denver, 1904.*

Principles of Teaching Special Subjects

25. Principles of Teaching Biology and Nature Study. *The Nature-Study Idea,* by L. H. Bailey, or *Nature Study and Life,* by C. F. Hodge, or *Nature Study for Common Schools,* by W. S. Jackman, or *The Teaching of Biology,* by F. E. Lloyd and M. E. Bigelow.

26. Principles of Teaching Chemistry and Physics. *The Teaching of Chemistry and Physics,* by A. Smith and E. H. Hall.

27. Principles of Teaching Domestic Science and Art. *The Teaching of Domestic Economy,* by H. Kinne, (announced for publication in 1906).

28. Principles of Teaching Drawing. *The Teaching of Drawing,* by I. H. Morris and *Composition,* by A. W. Dow.

29. Principles of Teaching English. *The Teaching of English,* by G. R. Carpenter, F. T. Baker and F. N. Scott, or *The Teaching of English,* by P. Chubb.

30. Principles of Teaching Geography. *The Teaching of Geography,* by A. Geikie, and either *Special*

278 · The Principles of Teaching

Method in Geography (edition of 1904 or later), by C. A. McMurry or *How to Study Geography*, by F. W. Parker or *The Teachers College Record*, vol. II. No. 2, by R. E. Dodge and C. B. Kirchwey.

31. Principles of Teaching History. *The Teaching of History and Civics*, by H. E. Bourne, or *Method in History*, by W. H. Mace, (1902 or later) or *Special Method in History*, by C. A. McMurry.

32. Principles of Teaching Latin and Greek. *The Teaching of Latin and Greek*, by C. E. Bennett and G. P. Bristol.   ·

33. Principles of Teaching Manual Art and Construction. *The Teaching of Manual Training*, by C. R. Richards, (announced for publication in 1906), or *The Teachers College Record*, vol. I, No. 5 and vol. II, No. 5, by C. R. Richards, A. V. Churchill, M. S. Woolman, H. Kinne and L. Rouillion.

34. Principles of Teaching Mathematics. *The Teaching of Elementary Mathematics*, by D. E. Smith.

35. Principles of Teaching Modern Languages. *New Methods of Teaching Modern Languages*, in the Teachers College Record, vol. IV, No. 3, by L. Bahlsen (translated by M. B. Evans), or *German in Secondary Schools*, by E. W. Bagster-Collins.

36. Principles of Teaching Music. *Music in the Schools*, by C. H. Farnsworth and M. Hofer, in the Teachers College Record, vol. V, No. 1, and the *Handbook on the Art of Teaching as Applied to Music*, by John Warriner.

37. Principles of Teaching Reading. *Reading, How to Teach It*, by S. L. Arnold and *Reading: A Manual for Teachers*, by M. E. Laing and *The Sentence Method of Teaching Reading* (1895 or later) by G. L. Farnham.

School Practices of the Past, and Reformers of Methods of Teaching

38. The Schools of Greece. *Elementary Greek Education*, by F. H. Lane and *Old Greek Education*, by J. P. Mahaffy.

Topics for Further Study   279

39. The Schools of Rome. *The Education of Children at Rome*, by G. Clarke.

40. The Schools of the Renaissance. *A Literary Source Book of the German Renaissance*, by M. Whitcomb (published by the Department of History of the University of Pennsylvania).

41. The Schools of England. *Schools, School-books and School-Masters*, by W. C. Hazlitt.

42. Comenius. *The Great Didactic*, edited by M. W. Keating, or *John Amos Comenius*, by S. S. Laurie, or *Comenius and the Beginnings of Educational Reform*, by W. S. Monroe and *The School of Infancy*, edited by W. S. Monroe.

43. Rousseau. *Émile*, Edited by W. H. Payne, or *Rousseau and Education According to Nature*, by T. Davidson.

44. Pestalozzi. *Pestalozzi*, by R. De Guimps, edited by J. Russell, or *Pestalozzi*, by A. Pinloche.

45. Herbart. *Herbart and the Herbartians*, by C. De Garmo.

46. Froebel. *Froebel and Education through Self-Activity*, by H. C. Bowen.

47. Stanley Hall. Chapters III, XII, XIII, XV and XVI of *Adolescence*, by G. Stanley Hall.

48. The Historical Course of Reform. *Essays on Educational Reformers*, by R. H. Quick (1890 or later).

49. American Education To-day. *Education in the United States*, edited by N. M. Butler (Albany, 1900).

BIBLIOGRAPHIES OF EDUCATION

The English-reading student will find the following sources of information about books on teaching sufficient:—For ordinary purposes, the *Bibliography of Education* by W. S. Monroe (1897) and the Bibliographies printed annually since 1900 in the *Educational Review* (New York). In addition, the Bibliographies of Child

280   *The Principles of Teaching*

Study printed annually in the *Pedagogical Seminary,* the *Analytical Index to the Educational Review,* vols. 1-25, by C. A. Nelson (1904) and *A Bibliography of Secondary Education,* by G. H. Locke (1903) may be consulted, and, of course, the indexes to general periodical literature.

THE SOURCES OF QUOTATIONS

1. W. JAMES, *Talks to Teachers on Psychology*, p. 62.
2. J. MACCUNN, *The Making of Character*, p. 29.
3. A. BAIN, *Education as a Science*, p. 90.
4. E. A. KIRKPATRICK, *Fundamentals of Child Study*, p. 208.
5. J. MACCUNN, *The Making of Character*, p. 10.
6. J. MACCUNN, *The Making of Character*, p. 29.
7. G. COMPAYRÉ, *Lectures on Pedagogy* (translated by Payne), 1890, p. 26.
8. P. A. BARNETT, *Common Sense in Education and Teaching*, p. 39.
9. The opening lines of the *Trimetrical Classic* of the Chinese.
10. E. A. KIRKPATRICK, *Fundamentals of Child Study*, p. 105.
11. F. FROEBEL, *Education of Man* (Hailmann's Translation), I, 8.
12. KIDDLE, HARRISON AND CALKINS, *How to Teach*, p. 17.
13. C. GUILLET, *Pedagogical Seminary*, Vol. VII, p. 427.
14. C. GUILLET, *Pedagogical Seminary*, Vol. VII, p. 445.
15. HARRIS, RICKOFF AND BAILEY, *Appleton's Second Reader*, (1878), pp. 8 and 9.
16. J. BALDWIN, *Industrial Primary Arithmetic*, p. 4.
17. J. DEWEY, *The Child and the Curriculum*, p. 38.
18. W. JAMES, *Talks to Teachers on Psychology*, p. 92.
19. M. H. CARTER, *The Kindergarten Child—After the Kindergarten, Atlantic Monthly*, March, 1899.

282   *The Principles of Teaching*

20. E. M. Cyr, *The Children's Second Reader*, (1894), (1897), pp. 92-97.

21. J. Baldwin, *School Reading by Grades*, Third Year, (1897), pp. 92-97.

22. Harris, Rickoff and Bailey, *Appleton's Second Reader*, (1878), p. 31.

23. E. C. Wilson, *Pedagogues and Parents*, p. 68.

24. J. M. Greenwood, *Principles of Education Practically Applied*, p. 27.

25. E. Lamborn, *The Practical Teacher*, p. 24.

26. P. P. G., *Exercises in Orthography*, p. 1 (so marked, though the following page is marked 6).

27. W. B. Fowle, *The Companion to Spelling Books*, p. 128.

28. R. Gilmour, *Second Reader of the Catholic National Series*, pp. 8-9.

29. *The Progressive Practical Arithmetic.*

30. J. Swett, *Examination Questions.*

31. J. Menet, *Practical Hints on Teaching*, p. 102.

32. J. Menet, *Practical Hints on Teaching*, p. 103.

33. *Infant School Manual*, quoted by S. R. Hall, *The Instructor's Manual*, p. 156.

34. Theodore Roosevelt.

35. W. James, *Talks to Teachers on Psychology*, pp. 68, 69.

36. From an advertisement of the Charles Field Street Academy (1826).

37. H. W. Ellsworth, *Text-book on Penmanship*, (1865), p. 140.

38. W. B. Fowle, *The Companion to Spelling Books*, p. 53.

39. W. B. Fowle, *The Companion to Spelling Books*, p. 83.

40. D. Putnam, *A Manual of Pedagogics*, p. 164.

The Sources of Quotations   283

41. W. JAMES (the author is unable to find the place where the anecdote appears in print, if indeed it is in print).

42. H. CREW, *Elements of Physics,* (1899), pp. 179-181.

43. H. A. AIKINS, *The Principles of Logic,* (1902), p. 31.

44. C. G. BURNHAM, *A New System of Arithmetic,* (1856), p. 17.

45. C. G. BURNHAM, *A New System of Arithmetic,* p. 243.

46. C. G. BURNHAM, *A New System of Arithmetic,* p. 271.

47. C. G. BURNHAM, *A New System of Arithmetic,* p. 23.

48. W. W. BEMAN AND D. E. SMITH, *Elements of Algebra,* (1901), p. 4.

49. W. W. BEMAN AND D. E. SMITH, *Elements of Algebra,* p. 41.

50. H. CREW, *Elements of Physics,* p. 19.

51. I. SHARPLESS AND G. M. PHILIPS, *Natural Philosophy,* (Revised Edition), p. 20.

52. H. CREW, *Elements of Physics,* p. 48.

53. I. SHARPLESS AND G. M. PHILIPS, *Natural Philosophy* (Revised Edition), p. 12.

54. H. G. BUEHLER, *A Modern English Grammar,* p. 207.

55. H. G. BUEHLER, *A Modern English Grammar,* p. 143.

56. E. POND, *Murray's System of English Grammar,* pp. 44-45.

57. G. J. SMITH, *Longman's English Grammar,* p. 159.

58. J. L. COMSTOCK, *A System of Natural Philosophy,* pp. 17-18.

59. L. D. HIGGINS, *Lessons in Physics,* pp. 19-21.

60. E. L. THORNDIKE, *Elements of Psychology,* pp. 293-294.

284 *The Principles of Teaching*

61. J. G. Fitch, *Lectures on Teaching*, p. 108.
62. J. G. Fitch, *Lectures on Teaching*, p. 109.
63. W. James, *Talks to Teachers on Psychology*, pp. 184, 185.
64. W. James, *Talks to Teachers on Psychology*, p. 71.
65. A. Smith, *Moral Sentiments*, VI, 3. (Quoted by J. MacCunn, in *The Making of Character*, p. 14.)
66. J. M. Greenwood, *Principles of Education Practically Applied*, p. 128.
67. H. C. Spencer, *Spencerian Key to Practical Penmanship*, (1869), p. 109.
68. H. Gordon, *Handwriting and How to Teach It*, p. 84.
69. H. Gordon, *Handwriting and How to Teach It*, p. 85.
70. H. C. Spencer, *Spencerian Key to Practical Penmanship*, p. 125.
71. H. C. Spencer, *Spencerian Key to Practical Penmanship*, p. 130.
72. H. C. Spencer, *Spencerian Key to Practical Penmanship*, pp. 131-132.
73. H. W. Ellsworth, *Text Book on Penmanship*, pp. 44-46.
74. Crosby and Nichols (?), *Theory and Art of Penmanship*, pp. 137-138.
75. A. T. Smith, *Systematic Methodology*, p. 202.
76. *Independent Fourth Reader*, p. 19 and p. 13.
77. E. L. Thorndike, *Educational Psychology* (1903), pp. 84-85.
78. W. C. Bagley, *The Educative Process*, p. 208.
79. N. Butler, quoted by E. L. Thorndike, *Educational Psychology*, p. 84.
80. W. Wilson, *Science*, Nov. 7, 1902.
81. E. H. Babbitt, in *Methods of Teaching Modern*

The Sources of Quotations 285

Languages, p. 130.

82. R. WORMELL, in *Teaching and Organization,* edited by P. A. BARNETT, p. 78.

83. C. THOMAS, in *Methods of Teaching Modern Languages,* p. 27. .

84. J. PAYNE, *Lectures on Education,* Vol. I, p. 261.

85. W. C. BAGLEY, *The Educative Process,* pp. 215-216.

86. J. PAYNE, *Lectures on Education,* Vol. I, p. 264.

87. J. ADAMS, *Herbartian Psychology Applied to Education,* p. 126.

88. I. H. MORRIS, in *Teaching and Organization,* edited by P. A. BARNETT, pp. 63-64.

89. J. PAYNE, *Lectures on Education,* Vol. I, p. 260.

90. D. PUTNAM, *A Manual of Pedagogics,* p. 243.

91. R. N. ROARK, *Method in Education,* p. 27.

92. E. H. BABBITT, in *Methods of Teaching Modern Languages,* p. 126

93. E. L. THORNDIKE and R. S. WOODWORTH, *Psychological Review,* Vol. VIII, pp. 249-250.

94. O. P. CORNMAN, *Spelling in the Elementary School,* pp. 47-48. , ,

95. O. P. CORNMAN, *Spelling in the Elementary School,* p. 59.

96. O. P. CORNMAN, *Spelling in the Elementary School,* pp. 62-63.

97. O. P. CORNMAN, *Spelling in the Elementary School,* pp. 69-70.

INDEX

Index of Exercises Relating to Special School Subjects

The references given are to the section and the number of the exercise. The number of the section is printed in italics; the number of the exercise in Roman.

Algebra.—§ *25*, 5; § *33*, 6; § *35*, 16; § *52*, 9; § *60*, 4.

Arithmetic.—§ *11*, 23; § *14*, 23, 30; § *18*, 26; § *25*, 5, Ex. 8; § *29*, 26, 27, 28, 29, 30, 37, 50; § *33*, 1, 2; § *35*, 19, 32; § *39*, 32, 33, 34, 35, 43, 44; § *52*, 9, 11; § *60*, 4, 7, 9, 10, 11.

Chemistry.—§ *14*, 24; § *18*, 7, 8; § *33*, 5; § *35*, 21, 28; § *39*, 21.

Drawing.—§ *18*, 6, Ex. 5; § *33*, 6; § *52*, 1, 2, 3, 4, 6, 9, 10; § *60*, 6.

English Composition.—§ *18*, 9, 24; § *33*, 5, 9

English Grammar.—§*3*, 2; §*14*, 11; § *25*, 5; § *29*, 34; § *35*, 2, 17, 32; § *39*, 14, 22, 23, 24, 25, 26, 29, 30, 31.

English Language.—§ *14*, 16; § *25*, 3; § *29*, 1, 2, 3, 4, 38.

English Literature. — § *3*, 1; § *18*, 12, 19; § *33*, 3, 9; § *47*, 6, 12; § *60*, 9. *See also under Reading.*

French.—§ *60*, 4.

Geography.—§ *3*, 8, 9; § *11*, 15, 21; § *14*, 5, 8, 22; § *31*, 5; § *33*, 6; § *39*, 14, 21; § *60*, 10, 11.

Geometry.—§ *11*, 20; § *18*, 27; § *29*, 47; § *35*, 3, 4, 5, 6, 7, 8, 13, 14, 15; § *39*, 7, 14, 36, 37, 38, 39, 40, 41, 42; § *60*, 4, 9, 12, 13, 14.

German.—§ *18*, 4; § *25*, 4; § *39*, 15; § *60*, 4, 6.

Greek.—§ *18*, 22; § *60*, 4, 5.

History.—§ *3*, 2; § *11*, 15, 22; § *14*, 9, 10, 21; § *18*, 4, 25; § *29*, 36; § *31*, 5; § *33*, 3, 6; § *47*, 7; § *52*, 9, 11.

Latin.—§ *3*, 1; § *18*, 28; § *25*, 4; § *29*, 7, 35; § *33*, 4; § *39*, 7, 21; § *52*, 9, 12; § *60*, 4, 5, 6, 9.

Manual Training.—§ *3*, 1; § *11*, 9; § *33*, 1.

Music.—§ *3*, 2; § *33*, 9.

Nature Study.—§ *11*, 9; § *14*, 25; § *18*, 30; § *35*, 31; § *39*, 27; § *47*, 9; § *52*, 11; § *60*, 15, 16, 17, 18.

Physics.—§ *35*, 22, 25, 29, 30, 32; § *39*, 15, 21, 28, 46, 47, 48; § *60*, 9, 12, 13, 14.

Physiology.—§ *14*, 26; § *18*, 22; § *52*, 9; § *60*, 12, 13.

Reading.—§ *7*, 10, Ex. 1; § *11*, 2; § *18*, 13, 15, 25, Ex. 7; § *29*, 6, 14, 15, 16, 17, 18, 19, 20, 21, 22, 23, 24; § *35*, 9, 10, 11, 12, 18, 27; § *52*, 9; § *55*, 6, 7.

286

Science.—§ *11*, 20; § *14*, 22, 28, 29; § *18*, 21; § *33*, 1, 6; § *39*, 45; § *60*, 6, 14, 15, 16, 17, 18.

Spelling.—§ *14*, 7; § *27*, 7, 8; § *29*, 5, 8; § *33*, 9. Writing.—§ *11*, 2; § *29*, 25; § *55*, 1, 2, 3, 4, 5.

INDEX OF EXPERIMENTS

1. The Influence of spacing upon the speed and ease of reading 19
2. Apperception: the over-estimation of children's knowledge 44
3 and 4. Apperception: city and country children compared 45
5. The interest of young children in drawing.............. 63
6. The interests of boys in their 'teens as shown by their reading 63
7. The interests of young children as shown by their preferences amongst reading lessons...................... 64
8. Individual differences in intellect...................... 98
9. Individual differences in taste........................ 101
10. The variability of the sexes........................... 104
11. Attention 108
12 and 13. The principles of association.................... 122
14. The inadequacy of practice without selection............ 231
15 and 16. The influence of special training on more general abilities 253-254

INDEX OF SUBJECTS

(The names of authors quoted in the text are also listed here.)

Abstraction (*See* Analysis).

Abstract thought, capacity for, 31 f.; interest in, 57 f.; individual differences in, 88; expression of by language, 209 f.

Accuracy in judging lengths and weights, 239, 241.

Action, children of, 86 f.; individual differences in, 92 ff.

Activity, instinct of physical, 25; instinct of mental, 26; self, 39 ff.; law of partial, 147, 153.

Adaptation of instruction to individual differences (*See* Individual differences).

Addition, individual differences in, 69 ff.

Adenoids, 15.

Aesthetic education, Chapter XII.

Aims of education, 3 ff.; variation of with conditions, 5 f.

Algebra, individual differences in, 81 f.

Analysis, as the basis of the higher mental activities, 133 f.; principles of teaching with respect to, Chapter IX; use of in teaching reasoning, 147 ff., 152 f., 155; exercises on, 135 ff.

Apperception, Chapter IV; and attention, 107; in motor education, 224 f.

Art, teaching of (*See* Motor expression and Motor education).

Association, individual differences in, 74 f.; principles of teaching with respect to, Chapter VIII; habit formation and, 110 ff.; memory and, 123 f.; systems of knowledge and, 127 ff.; exercises on, 112 ff.

Athletics, and moral training, 185.

Attention, Chapter VII; caused by instincts and habits, 105; gaining *vs.* holding, 106; influence of bodily attitudes on, 106 f.; in motor education, 226; influence of special training of, 241; exercises on, 107 ff.

Attitude, instincts of, 24 (*See* also Physical Attitudes).

BAGLEY, W. C., 242.

BENNETT, C., 240.

BENSON, A. C., 187.

Bodily (*See* Physical).

Body, influence of on mind, 13 f.

Index

289

Capacities, Chapter III; development of, 21; inhibition of, 21 f.; delayed, 22; individual differences in, 23 f., 32 f.; important in school life, 30; for abstract thought, 31 f.; for managing ideas, 31; for cooperation, 32; for leadership, 32; for originality and self-reliance, 32; neglect of, 32; specialization of, 33, 238 ff.; exercises on, 34 ff.

Classes, size of, in relation to moral training, 184; in relation to methods of instruction (See Individual differences).

Classification, of responses, 9; of stimuli, 8.

Collecting, instinct of, 27.

Comparison, as an aid in teaching analysis, 135; in teaching reasoning, 151 f., 156 f.

Conduct (*See* Moral training).

Contrast, as an aid in teaching reasoning, 151 f., 156 f.

Cooperation, capacity for, 32.

CORNMAN, O. P., 268 ff.

Correlation, 127 ff.; means of securing, 128; danger to be avoided in, 129; exercises on, 129 ff.

Deduction, 154 f. (*See* also Deductive).

Deductive methods of teaching, 160 ff.; difficulties in, 160; selection of essential elements in, 161 f.; means of guidance in, 163 f.; exercises on, 164 ff.

Defects, physical, 14; of intellect, 88 f.

Definitions, use of in analysis, 135.

Delayed capacities and instincts, 22; in relation to motor education, 223 f.

Development, of instincts and capacities, 21; of interests, 52 f.; of motor ability, 223 f.

DEWEY, J., 56.

Differences, between individuals (*See* Individual differences); between the sexes (*See* Sex differences).

Discipline, formal (*See* Formal discipline); moral training and school, 186 f.

Dissociation (*See* Analysis).

Distribution of mental abilities, 68 ff.

Drawing (*See* Motor expression and Motor education).

Drill in spelling, apparent futility of, 268 ff.

Education (*See* specific headings).

Elements, analysis of, 133 ff.; selection of in reasoning, 148 ff., 161 ff.

Emotions, education of the, Chapter XII.

Ethical training (*See* Moral training).

Examinations (*See* Testing).

Execution, teaching of in the motor arts, 222 ff.

Exercise of the muscles, 12 f.

Expression (*See* Motor expression).

290 *Index*

Faculty psychology (*See* Formal discipline).

Feeling, children of, 86; responses of, Chapter XII.

Feelings, education of the, Chapter XII; association and, 199; bodily attitudes and, 199 f.; imitation and, 199; in the case of the aesthetic feelings, 201 f.; exercises on, 202 ff.

Form, teaching of in the motor arts, 220 f.

Formal discipline, Chapter XV; meaning of, 235 f.; common view of, 236 f.; inconsistent with the specialization of abilities, 238 ff.; amount of, 240 ff.; in sense-training, 240; in observation and attention, 241; in memory, 241; in neatness, 242; methods of securing, 243 ff.; exercises on, 249 ff.

Formal steps of instruction, 159 f.

Fracker, G. C., 241.

Geography and moral training, 190 f.

Gilbert, J. A., 241.

Gymnastics, 12 f.

Habit, Chapter VIII; and attention, 105; and the education of the feelings, 199.

Health, Chapter II.

Hearing, defects of, 14.

History and moral training, 191 f.

Hygiene (*See* Physical education).

Identical elements, disciplinary effect through, 243 ff.

Imagery, applications to teaching of individual differences in, 89 ff.

Imitation, 25, 53, 184, 199, 220 f.

Improvement of general powers (*See* Formal discipline).

Inattention, 105.

Inborn tendencies (*See* Instincts and Capacities).

Incentives (See Interests).

Individual differences, Chapter VI; in instincts and capacities, 23 f.; nature, 68 f.; distribution of, 68 ff.; amount, 69 ff.; range, 72 ff.; concrete illustrations of, 76 ff.; in addition, 69 ff.; in rate of movement, 73; in observation, 74 f.; in association, 74 f.; in spelling, 74 f., 83; in logical power, 76 f.; in memory, 78 f.; in ability to translate Latin, 79 f.; in algebra, 81 f.; pedagogical consequences of, 83 ff.; in general mental constitution, 85 ff.; in thought, 87 ff.; in imagery, 89 ff.; in action, 92 ff.; in suggestibility, 94; in temperament, 94 ff.; exercises on, 98 ff.

Induction (See Inductive).

Inductive methods of teaching, 154 ff.; verification in, 157 f.; use of types in, 158 f.; formal steps of instruction in, 159 f.

Index

291

Inhibition, of instincts and capacities, 21 f.; and self activity, 40; of interests, 52.

Instincts, Chapter III; meaning of to teaching, 21 f.; delayed, 22; transitory, 22; individual differences in, 23 f.; of attitude, 24; of mental activity, 25; of physical activity, 26; of collecting, 27; of pugnacity, 27; neglect of in teaching, 27 f.; misuse of, 28 f.; and attention, 105; and moral training, 182; and the training of the emotions, 198 f.; exercises on, 34 ff.

Intellect, types of, 87 f.; defectives in, 88 f. (*See* also Reasoning).

Interests, Chapter V; instinctive, 24; as ends of teaching, 51 ff.; as means, 54 ff.; native, 52; acquired, 52; inhibition of, 52; development of, 52 f.; habit and, 53; imitation and, 53; knowledge and, 53; essential in teaching, 54 ff.; and difficulty, 56 f.; and pleasure, 57; in abstract thought, 57 f.; must be in the right thing, 58; and expression through material constructions, 211 f.; exercises on, 59 ff.

JAMES, W., 29, 121.

Language, as a means of expression, 208 ff.

Latin, individual differences in, 79 f.

Leadership, capacity for, 32.

Limitations to teaching reasoning, 153 f.; to moral training, 180 ff., 184 f.

Literature and moral training, 191 f.

Logical thinking (*See* Reasoning); individual differences in, 76 f.

Material constructions as means of expression, 210 ff.

Material of education, 7 ff.

MacCunn, J., 29.

Memory, 123 ff.; individual differences in, 78 f.; influence of special training of, 241; exercises on, 124 ff.

Mental balance, 95.

Methods, of education, 6; of influence of special training on general ability, 243 ff; tests of, 264 ff.

Mind, influence of the body on, 13 f.

Moral training, Chapter XI; analysis of, 179 f.; limitations to in schools, 180 ff., 184 f.; instincts in, 182; association in, 182; partial activity in, 182; suggestion in, 183; school habits and, 185; school discipline and, 186 f.; specific lessons in, 187 ff.; ordinary studies and, 189 ff.; geography as, 190 f.; history and literature as, 191 f.; exercises on, 194 ff.

Motor education, Chapter XIV; equals teaching form and teaching execution,

292 *Index*

219 f.; principles of teaching form in, 220 f.; imitation in, 221; principles of teaching execution in, 222 ff.; selection by resultant satisfaction in, 222; delayed capacities and, 223 f.; apperception in, 224 f.; attention in, 226; self criticism by pupils, 226 f.; exercises on, 228 ff.

Motor expression, Chapter XIII; need of in teaching, 206; varieties of, 207 f.; verbal expression, 208 ff.; the activities of the arts and industries in, 210 ff.; dangers to be avoided in, 212 ff.; exercises on, 215 ff.

Movement (*See* motor); individual differences in rate of, 73.

Muscles (*See* motor); exercise of, 12 f.

Natural tendencies (*See* Instincts and Capacities).

Neatness, influence of special training in, 242.

Normal children, 68 ff.

Object lessons, 48.

Observation, individual differences in, 74 f.; influence of special training in, 241.

PARKER and HASWELL, 158.

Partial activity, the law of in teaching reasoning, 147; in moral training, 182.

Physical activity, instinct of, 25;

not equivalent to self-activity, 40.

Physical attitudes, influence of on attention, 106 f.; on responses of feeling, 199 f.

Physical defects, 14 ff.; remedying, 14 f.; prevention, 16 f.

Physical education, Chapter II; as an end, 12 f.; as a means, 13 f.; exercises, 17 ff.

Pleasure, and interests, 57.

Powers, training of the mental (*See* Formal discipline).

Process of education, 1.

Psychology and teaching, 7 ff.

Pugnacity, 27.

Range of individual differences, 72 ff.

Realism in teaching, 48.

Reasoning, Chapter X; as selective thinking, 147 ff.; the abstraction of elements as a feature of, 147 ff., 155; verification as a feature of, 148 f., 157 f.; difficulties in teaching, 150 f.; comparison and contrast as aids in, 151 f.; induction and deduction, 154 f.; principles of teaching inductions, 156 ff.; use of types in teaching, 158 f.; formal steps of instruction in, 159 f.; principles of teaching deductions, 160 ff.; difficulties in, 160 f.; adaptation of to capacities, 163 f.; exercises on, 164 ff.

Reliance, self, capacity for, 32.

Responses, classification of, 9.

Index

293

Results of teaching (*See* Testing).

Results of different methods (*See* Testing).

RICE, J. M., 269.

School hygiene (*See* Physical education).

Scientific study of teaching, Chapter XVI.

Selection, in teaching reasoning, 147 ff.

Self-activity, 39 ff.; bodily activity and, 40; inhibition and, 40.

Self-reliance, capacity for, 32.

Sense discrimination, influence of special training in, 240.

Sex differences, 96 f.; in type, 96; in variability, 96 f.

Sight, defects of, 14 f.

Skill (*See* Motor education).

SMITH, ADAM, 199.

Special training, influence of on general ability (*See* Formal discipline).

Specialization of abilities, 33, 238 ff.

Spelling, individual differences in, 74 f., 83; scientific study of, 268 ff.

SQUIRE, C. G., 242.

Steps of instruction, formal, 159 f.

Stimuli, classification of, 8.

Suggestibility, individual differences in, 94.

Suggestion as a means of moral training, 183.

Teachers, relation of to higher educational authorities, 1 ff., 6.

Teaching (*See* under specific headings such as Apperception, Attention, Interest).

Temperament, 94 ff.

Testing the results of methods, 264 ff.; need of science in, 265 ff.; the duty of educational leaders, 267 f.; a sample of scientific procedure in, 268 ff.

Testing the results of particular acts of teaching, 257 ff.; importance of, 257 f.; difficulty of, 258 f., 260; value of, 259; rules for, 260 ff.

THORNDIKE, E. L., 180, 241.

Thought, children of, 85 f.; individual differences in, 87 ff.

Tonsils enlarged, 15.

Training of mental powers (*See* Formal discipline).

Types, as central tendencies, 71; of general mental constitution, 85 ff.; of intellect, 87 ff.; of will, 92 ff.; of temperament, 94 ff.; use of in teaching inductions, 158 f.

Variability, 68 ff.; of the sexes, 96 f.

Verification as a feature of teaching reasoning, 148 ff., 157 f.

Vision (*See* Sight).

Will, types of, 92 ff.

WOODWORTH, R. S., 241.

CPSIA information can be obtained
at www.ICGtesting.com
Printed in the USA
BVHW062315080319
542203BV00009B/92/P